Outdoor Firs

C000279403

Outdoor First Aid is published by: **Nuco Training Ltd**

WHAT IS OUTDOOR FIRST AID?

First aid saves lives, and knowing what to do in an outdoor emergency situation will make a significant difference when helping someone who is sick or injured. There are many environmental factors to consider in an outdoor setting and this book will provide you with the knowledge and skills to administer first aid effectively where it may prove challenging for the emergency services to reach you in a short period of time.

Outdoor First Aid procedures may be needed for activities such as hiking, running, camping, cycling, climbing or any activity that takes place outside in the open air, that is distant from the emergency services.

DEFINITION OF FIRST AID

First aid is the initial treatment given to someone who is injured or sick, prior to professional medical assistance arriving and taking over from you.

AIMS OF FIRST AID

As a First Aider, your priorities for the casualty fall into the following categories:

PRESERVE life

ALLEVIATE suffering

PREVENT further illness or injury

PROMOTE recovery

For example, if your casualty has fallen onto a jagged rock and cuts their arm, you can preserve life by offering treatment immediately and not waiting for professional help to sort it out for you. If you do nothing, your casualty could bleed to death. We can alleviate suffering by making the casualty more comfortable, keeping them warm and offering lots of care and attention. We can prevent further illness or injury by applying a secure sterile dressing over the wound in order to control the blood loss and prevent the risk of infection.

We can promote recovery by treating the casualty for shock and summoning for professional medical assistance as soon as possible.

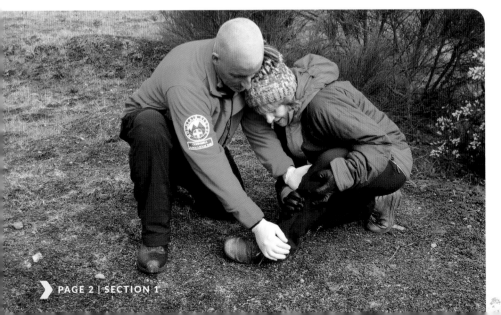

HOW OUTDOOR FIRST AID IS DIFFERENT

In an urban setting, we rely heavily on medical professionals to provide assistance when someone falls sick or becomes injured. In most cases, help arrives very quickly, equipped with the necessary resources to aid the casualty and to keep them alive and well. Although the protocols and procedures are comparable to that of First Aid at Work, Outdoor First Aid has a more distinct focus, because:

- **Illnesses and injuries occur outdoors, often in adverse conditions that affect both the casualty and the rescuer**
- **Professional medical assistance may be delayed for extended periods of time due to difficult locations, severe weather conditions and a lack of communication and transportation**
- **Certain injuries and illnesses are far more common in remote locations** (sprains and strains, frostbite, insect stings, blisters, hypothermia)
- **First aid supplies and equipment may be limited**
- **Important decisions must be made. For example: Deciding whether to move and evacuate your casualty**

FIRST AID KITS, CONTAINERS AND CONTENTS

Before venturing into the outdoor environment, whether you are hiking, cycling, running or similar, you must ensure that you are appropriately prepared with first aid and survival equipment. This will vary from person to person depending on the individual circumstances and the activity taking place.

There is no mandatory list of items to be included in a first aid container, and that also applies to Outdoor First Aid. In the workplace, the decision on what to provide will depend on the outcome of the risk assessment of first aid needs. Deciding what to pack for the outdoor environment will also need careful consideration and planning.

You will need to perform your own 'risk assessment', considering the risk factors attached to the activities and the possible injuries or illnesses that are likely to occur.

You can use any type of container to hold your first aid supplies, but you should consider:

The material   is the container weatherproof, durable and easy to recognise?

The size   will the container fit in your rucksack or in a suitable compartment?

The shape   is the shape of the container suitable and easy to obtain in an emergency?

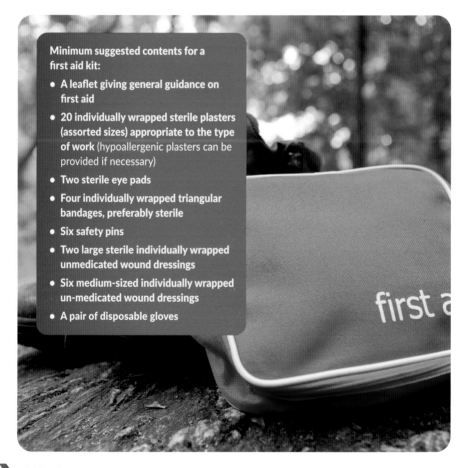

Minimum suggested contents for a first aid kit:

- **A leaflet giving general guidance on first aid**

- **20 individually wrapped sterile plasters (assorted sizes) appropriate to the type of work** (hypoallergenic plasters can be provided if necessary)

- **Two sterile eye pads**

- **Four individually wrapped triangular bandages, preferably sterile**

- **Six safety pins**

- **Two large sterile individually wrapped unmedicated wound dressings**

- **Six medium-sized individually wrapped un-medicated wound dressings**

- **A pair of disposable gloves**

ADDITIONAL ITEMS THAT MAY PROVE USEFUL TO CARRY IN YOUR OUTDOOR FIRST AID KIT:

- Tweezers
- Face shields
- Tick removal tool
- Saline solution pods
- Scissors
- Clinical waste bags
- Burns dressings
- Haemostatic dressings
- Blister plasters

- Glucose tablets or gel
- Medical tape
- Tourniquets
- Survival blankets
- Antiseptic wipes
- Instant ice packs
- Medication
- Small torch

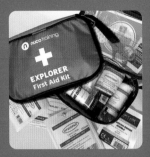

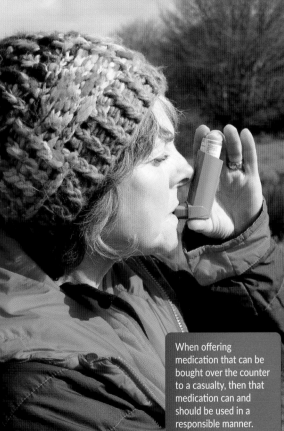

MEDICATION

It is recommended that medication and tablets should not be stored in a first aid kit. However, for the purposes of Outdoor First Aid, you may need to carry certain types of medication and tablets which could prove vital if an incident was to occur.

The medication does not have to be stored inside your first aid kit. This can be stored separately in a clearly labelled, individual bag. It would prove useful to have a copy of the dosage requirements and a list of any contraindications that apply to the medication.

Medication could include:

- Paracetamol
- Aspirin
- Ibuprofen
- Diarrhoea tablets
- Asthma inhaler (if asthmatic)
- Antihistamine

When offering medication that can be bought over the counter to a casualty, then that medication can and should be used in a responsible manner.

EMERGENCY SHELTERS

Emergency shelters are temporary structures that can be used for:

- **A general place of rest**
- **To protect yourself against the elements**
- **To 'preserve life' if someone falls sick or injured**

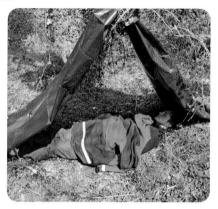

Shelters can also offer you protection from wildlife and airborne contaminants that may pose a risk.

Knowing how to create the most basic of shelters could make a significant difference in keeping your casualty alive, as well as yourself. Not only do temporary shelters help physical needs, but they also help to create a sense of home in an outdoor setting, which may benefit you and any casualty, alleviating any worries relating to the incident.

Fortunately, there are now many suppliers who offer purpose-built emergency shelters at reasonable prices that can be set-up in a matter of seconds, saving you a considerable amount of time and energy in an emergency situation.

Emergency shelters can include:

Bivouac sack (also known as a 'bivi bag')

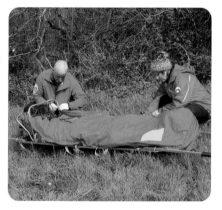

A thin, lightweight, waterproof bag that is designed to slip over a sleeping bag to retain body heat and provide additional insulation, forming a barrier against the elements.

One of the key benefits is the speed in which it can be set-up and the ability to use it in very small spaces. A disadvantage of a bivouac sack is the humidity that condenses on the inner side, leaving the occupant and/or the sleeping bag damp and moist. Bivouac sacks are usually designed for one person.

Bothy bag

Similar to the bivouac sack, a bothy bag is a lightweight portable emergency shelter that offers protection from the elements. Bothy bags come in a variety of sizes, ranging from a 2-person bag up to a 20-person bag. Tents can be very bulky to carry, but most bothy bags will fit comfortably in a large rucksack. To form the shelter, the sack is pulled out from its carry bag and then pulled over you and the group, forming a 'cocoon' like shelter. Bothy bags are usually large enough for the number of occupants it is designed for, plus additional space in the centre for eating, drinking and caring for a casualty.

CASUALTY REPORT FORM

A casualty report form is used to gather information about your casualty, which is then handed to the emergency services when they arrive and take over from you.

The form will be a useful point of reference when assessing your casualty and monitoring any vital signs. Casualty report forms come in a variety of formats, but all serve the same purpose.

The form will usually contain guidance notes next to each entry field as a reminder, and to ensure you complete the form accurately.

The casualty report form needs to stay with your casualty at all times and making sure the form leaves with the rescue services is paramount, as this gives them accurate information to continue caring for your casualty.

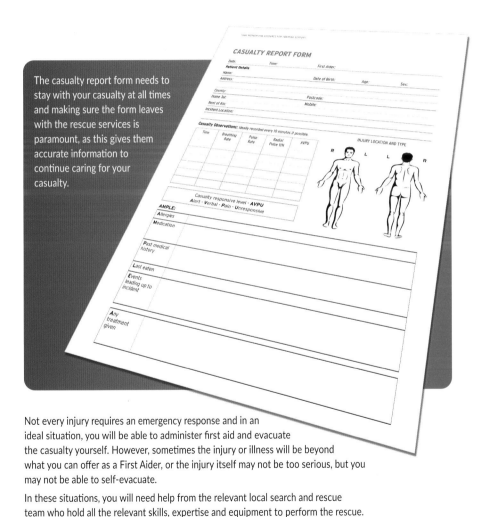

Not every injury requires an emergency response and in an ideal situation, you will be able to administer first aid and evacuate the casualty yourself. However, sometimes the injury or illness will be beyond what you can offer as a First Aider, or the injury itself may not be too serious, but you may not be able to self-evacuate.

In these situations, you will need help from the relevant local search and rescue team who hold all the relevant skills, expertise and equipment to perform the rescue. Search and rescue teams may use a search dog to track your location and even dispatch a helicopter to assist with the rescue.

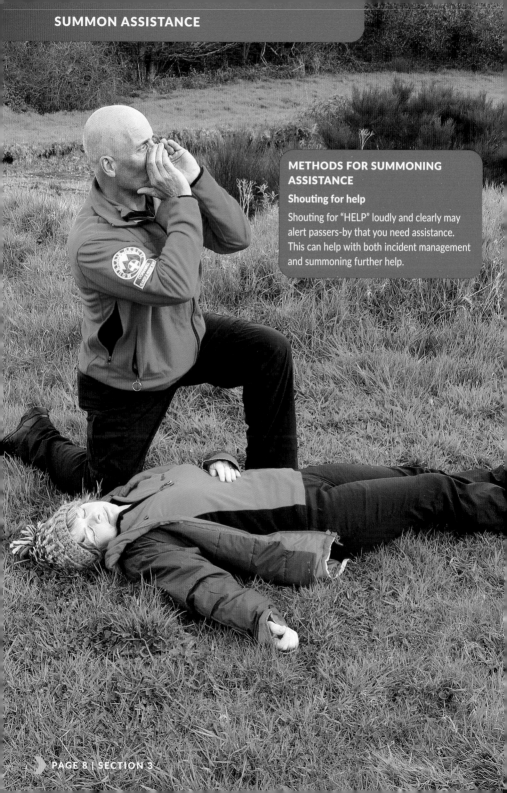

METHODS FOR SUMMONING ASSISTANCE

Shouting for help

Shouting for "HELP" loudly and clearly may alert passers-by that you need assistance. This can help with both incident management and summoning further help.

International Distress Signal

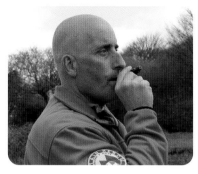

The International Distress Signal can be recognised by either 6 short blasts of a whistle, or 6 flashes of a light repeated every minute. This should be continued even if someone is replying, commonly with 3 blasts or 3 flashes every minute.

Morse code

Although very similar, Morse code differs to the International Distress Signal and can be recognised by a number of different means, i.e. Beeps on a radio, blasts of a whistle, flashes of a light, etc. It follows the same pattern: **3 short, 3 long, 3 short or ... _ _ _ ...**

Telephone / mobile phone

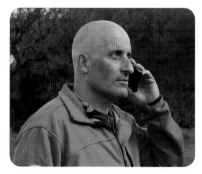

In remote locations, a mobile phone signal can be limited and a decision may have to be made about leaving your casualty in order to summon help. If the signal is an issue, consider any points where you may have had a signal, or a house where there may be a landline. If you have to use a landline and your casualty is not mobile, it will mean you have to leave them to make the call.

Where an incident has occurred in a remote location, access and egress is likely to be an issue. In this scenario, you will need to ask for "mountain rescue" to provide professional medical assistance.

Mountain rescue can be contacted by:

DIALLING 999/112, REQUESTING THE "POLICE" AND THEN ASKING FOR "MOUNTAIN RESCUE".

Often where there is little or no signal, a phone may still be able to connect, but it may have a message saying, "**SOS only**".

PLEASE NOTE:
Due to the dynamics of this subject, 'call the emergency services' will be used as generic term throughout this publication, covering all types of emergency service that you may require. When an incident occurs that requires professional help, common sense must prevail to determine which emergency service(s) are required, depending on the situation and your location.

If you are in any doubt, continue to **dial 999/112** and explain the situation to the operator.

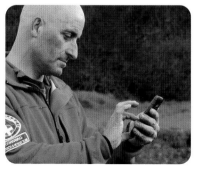

Text message

Sending a text message requires much less signal strength and the phone will keep trying to send the text for a short period of time meaning there is a greater chance of the message getting through if you are moving, or in an area of changeable reception.

EMERGENCYSMS SERVICE

In the UK, EmergencySMS is a simple and innovative system that was designed to aid people who are deaf or have a hearing or speech impairment to text the emergency services. It should be noted that a mobile phone must be registered with this service to use it.

To register:

1. Send the word 'register' in an SMS message to "**999**"
2. You will then receive SMS messages about the service
3. When you have read these SMS messages, reply by sending 'yes' in an SMS message to "**999**"
4. You will receive an SMS message telling you that your mobile phone is registered, or if there is a problem with your registration

If you try to register and do not receive an SMS message from the EmergencySMS service, please check with your mobile communications provider to make sure they support the EmergencySMS service.

Visit www.emergencysms.org.uk for more information.

PROCEDURE FOR MAKING AN EMERGENCY CALL

Before contacting the emergency services, make sure you have the following details to hand, as this is what you will be asked to provide:

- **Your location** (consider grid reference, GPS, landmarks, points of reference etc.)
- **What has happened and when**
- **Name, gender and age of casualty(s)**
- **Nature and extent of the injury or illness**
- **Number of people in the party and a description of clothing and colours worn**
- **Any significant hazards that the rescue services will need to be aware of**
- **Your name and mobile phone number** (and a reserve number if held)

    If you need to send a bystander to seek help for you, ensure that they have all the correct information to pass on and remind them to return as soon as possible.

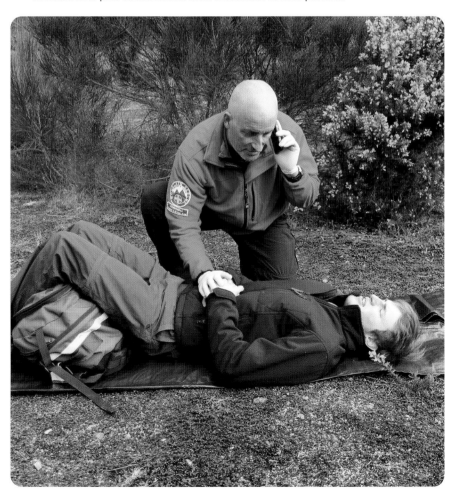

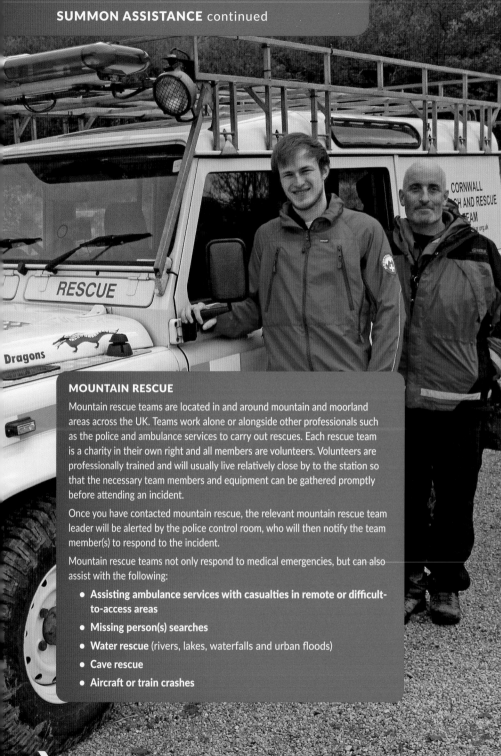

MOUNTAIN RESCUE

Mountain rescue teams are located in and around mountain and moorland areas across the UK. Teams work alone or alongside other professionals such as the police and ambulance services to carry out rescues. Each rescue team is a charity in their own right and all members are volunteers. Volunteers are professionally trained and will usually live relatively close by to the station so that the necessary team members and equipment can be gathered promptly before attending an incident.

Once you have contacted mountain rescue, the relevant mountain rescue team leader will be alerted by the police control room, who will then notify the team member(s) to respond to the incident.

Mountain rescue teams not only respond to medical emergencies, but can also assist with the following:

- **Assisting ambulance services with casualties in remote or difficult-to-access areas**
- **Missing person(s) searches**
- **Water rescue** (rivers, lakes, waterfalls and urban floods)
- **Cave rescue**
- **Aircraft or train crashes**

SEARCH DOGS

If you are unable to provide an accurate update on your location when making the emergency call, it is possible that mountain rescue will deploy a search dog to pin-point your location. In this type of situation, it is important to stay where you are with the casualty. Search dogs are trained to ignore moving people and follow the scent on the wind. It will then run between you and its handler in a back and forth motion until all three are united.

Training the dog can take as long as two years, as dog teams work through a series of grades and assessments before becoming fully qualified. Even as a fully-qualified search dog, training and assessment continues throughout a dog's working life. The majority of search dogs are Border Collies, although other breeds include the Labrador and German Shepherd.

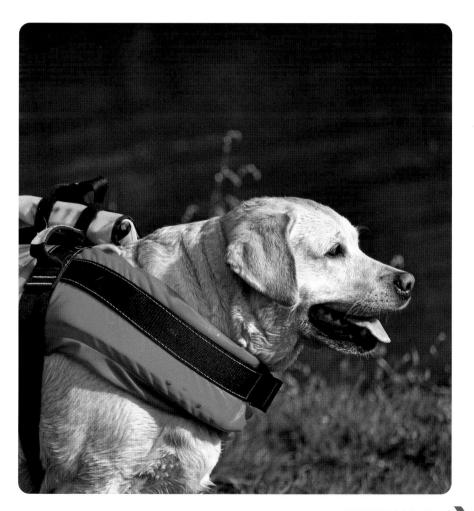

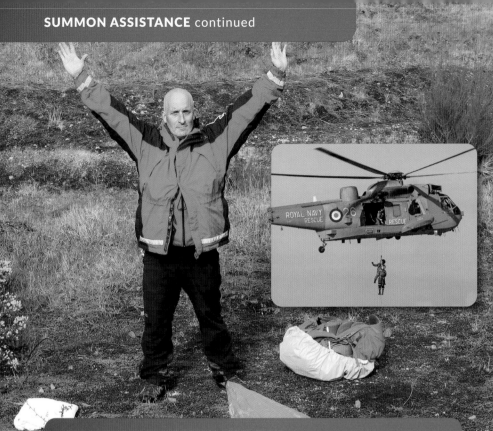

ATTRACTING A HELICOPTER'S ATTENTION

On occasions, it may prove difficult for the helicopter crew to actually distinguish who needs help if there are a number of people in the area. A helicopter will not be despatched automatically for each and every rescue, only when it is absolutely necessary. This is usually when someone has been critically injured or has suffered a life-threatening illness that requires immediate and specialist care. The correct way of attracting a helicopter's attention is not waving, yelling or jumping, but to stand still in a Y position with your feet together and arms open wide above your head. This can be assisted by laying out brightly coloured clothing or materials on the ground so that it is more visible from the air.

During night time, you are more likely to hear the helicopter before you can see it. This gives you a small amount of time to prepare and attract its attention. The most common methods of attracting a helicopter's attention at night-time are:

Torch

Pointed directly at the ground in a sweeping motion (*never shine the torch directly at the helicopter*).

Glow Stick

Spun round your head on a bit of string. It will make a very large easily visible 'O' shape.

If you do not have a torch or glow stick, it may be possible to use the light on the back of your mobile phone, or the flash from a camera to attract its attention.

MONITORING VITAL SIGNS

When treating your casualty, you will need to monitor their vital signs which will help you identify problems and indicate any changes to their condition. Vital signs are measurements of the body's most basic functions, which include:

- **Level of response**
- **Breathing**
- **Pulse**
- **Skin colour**
- **Body temperature**

Monitoring should be repeated at regular intervals and the information gathered should be handed over to the relevant emergency service when they arrive and take over from you. Ideally, the information you have gathered should be written down on a casualty report form. If you do not have this, a notepad or sheet of paper will be adequate.

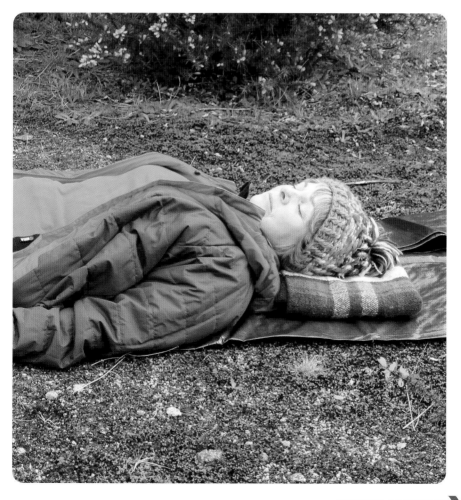

METHODS FOR MONITORING VITAL SIGNS

Ask your casualty leading questions which allow you to build up a history of progression and respond accordingly.

How do you feel? Is it getting worse? Is the pain spreading?

Breathing

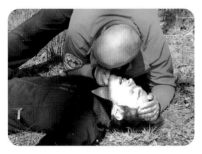

Monitor your casualty's breathing rate and note any changes. This could be difficult if they are wearing lots of layers, so you may have to consider other means to monitor without compromising the airway. The average adult will take 10-20 breaths per minute and the average child, between 20-30 breaths per minute. Babies are much more frequent with an average of 30-40 breaths per minute. As well as their respiration rate, you can listen for wheezing or gasping sounds - this is not normal breathing and you must commence CPR without delay.

Pulse

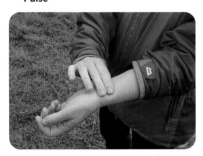

Use fingers and not the thumb to take their pulse. Record the rate in either the wrist or the neck in beats per minute, whether it is strong or weak and if it is a normal rhythm. A pulse level can be affected by someone's fitness or by medication they may be taking. An average adult could have a pulse of anything between 60-100 beats per minute. A pulse is not used to determine whether or not to proceed with CPR, it is only when the casualty is not breathing normally that you must commence CPR.

Skin colour

Light skinned people will appear pale, white, grey or ashen if circulation is poor. Lips, nails and in some instances, the skin may appear blue indicating low levels of oxygen in the blood. Detecting change to the skin in darker skinned people can be tricky. The best assessment is to check the lining of the mouth which should be flushed. If it is pale, or in some instances white, then it is an indication that their circulation is poor.

Body temperature

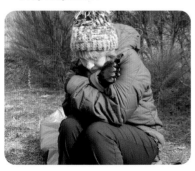

In the outdoor environment it may prove difficult to monitor the temperature of your casualty. If your casualty is responsive, the best method is questioning. However, casualties suffering with extreme hypothermia where they are very cold, may say they feel hot. Similarly, casualties with severe hyperthermia where they are too hot, may say they feel too cold.

RESPONDING TO A CHANGE IN VITAL SIGNS

Continuing with the activity

If your casualty wishes to continue with the activity, are they physically able to? What are the risks to both you and your casualty? If your casualty decides they would like to continue with the activity, you will need to monitor them carefully and re-assess the situation at regular intervals.

Evacuation

If your casualty cannot continue with the activity because the injury or illness has become too serious, you may need to self-evacuate. It may be possible for the casualty to walk themselves, or with you supporting them.

Equipment

What is on hand to deal with a change in signs and what are the implications for the rest of the group?

Making sure you have packed the relevant first aid supplies and equipment will be recognised and appreciated at this moment in time, as it could mean the difference in saving your casualty's life.

Moving an injured casualty

If your casualty cannot walk, care needs to be taken when self-evacuating. The safety to you and your casualty must remain paramount - never hesitate to re-assess the situation and call for help if your casualty's condition deteriorates, or you become too tired to continue.

Calling for help

The vital signs may change to the point where it is necessary to call for help. If the casualty is going to be left stationary whilst this happens, it is important to provide shelter and insulate the casualty from the ground. If you decide that professional help is necessary, dial 999/112 and request the relevant emergency service.

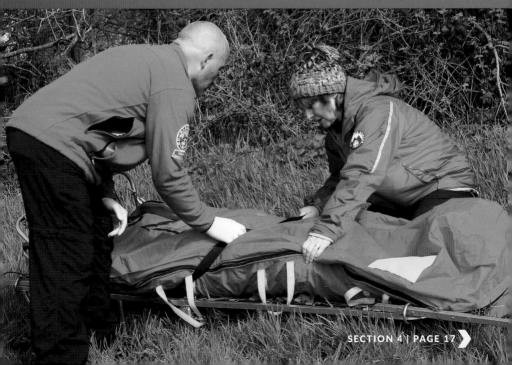

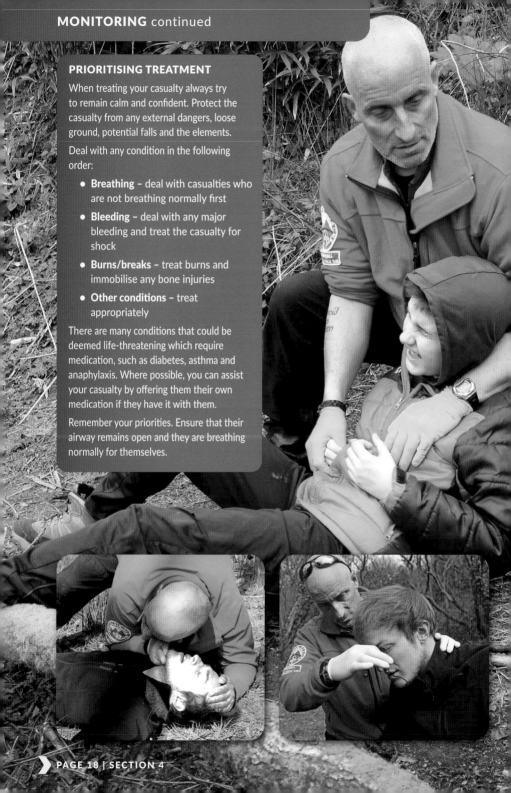

PRIORITISING TREATMENT

When treating your casualty always try to remain calm and confident. Protect the casualty from any external dangers, loose ground, potential falls and the elements.

Deal with any condition in the following order:

- **Breathing** – deal with casualties who are not breathing normally first
- **Bleeding** – deal with any major bleeding and treat the casualty for shock
- **Burns/breaks** – treat burns and immobilise any bone injuries
- **Other conditions** – treat appropriately

There are many conditions that could be deemed life-threatening which require medication, such as diabetes, asthma and anaphylaxis. Where possible, you can assist your casualty by offering them their own medication if they have it with them.

Remember your priorities. Ensure that their airway remains open and they are breathing normally for themselves.

CONDUCTING A SCENE SURVEY

A scene survey involves assessing the situation to work out what has happened, how and why, before moving on to the primary survey. The scene survey begins as soon as you realise that there is an emergency situation and may include:

Managing the incident

Keep calm and collected, try not to show panic. Act promptly but cautiously to ensure the safety of all. Look around at the scene to establish what has happened, and to make sure any on-lookers are kept well clear of the area.

Looking for potential hazards

Look around for anything that has the potential to cause harm to you, your casualty and any bystanders. Identifying hazards at this stage can prevent the risk of further casualties.

Outdoor hazards may include:

- **Adverse weather conditions** (lightning, snow, heavy rain)
- **Rough terrain, wet grass, wet rocks, greasy surfaces**
- **Moving people** (walkers, runners, cyclists, skiers, snowboarders)
- **Rockfalls & snowslides**
- **Flooding**
- **Falling trees**
- **Poisonous animals, plants and insects**
- **Sharp objects, holes and animal burrows**

Assessing the situation

Gather information from your casualty (if possible) and any bystanders at the scene. This may prove difficult if you are on your own with no bystanders available to assist you. Look for anything that may have caused the injury or illness and the current position of the casualty.

Protecting against contamination

Prevent cross-infection by wearing disposable gloves and only use sterile first aid supplies to treat your casualty. Make the most of any bystanders present which may include calling the emergency services, fetching first aid equipment and cordoning off the area.

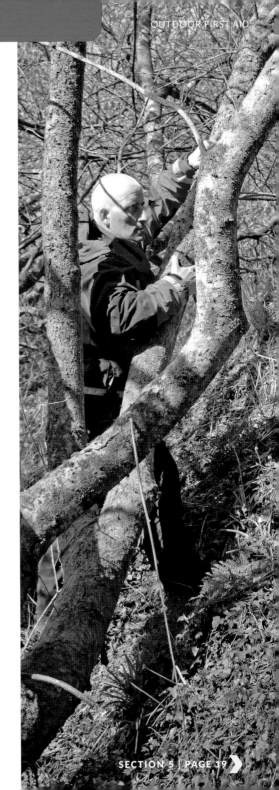

CONSENT

A responsive adult must agree to receive first aid treatment. Expressed consent means the casualty gives their permission to receive care and treatment. To obtain consent, first identify yourself, tell them about your level of training and qualification and ask if it's ok to help them.

Implied consent means that permission to perform first aid care on an unresponsive casualty is assumed. This is based on the idea that a reasonable person would give their permission to receive lifesaving treatment if they were able to.

CASUALTY COMMUNICATION

Irrespective of the severity of the incident, your casualty could be in a state of shock and confusion. Therefore, your communication skills are critical in gaining their trust.

- **Be honest about their condition, without exaggerating it**
- **Be careful of what you say which could distress them further and take your time when talking to them**
- **Try and maintain eye contact when talking to them and be aware of your body language. Their body language could tell you a lot about their condition**
- **Allow your casualty to explain how they are feeling** (if they are able to). **This could help you make a diagnosis enabling you to offer the right treatment**

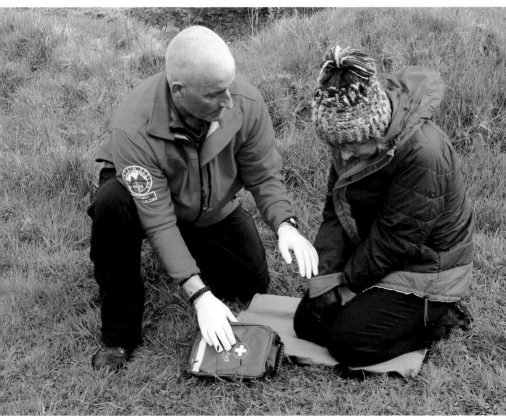

After the scene survey, you will need to move on to the initial assessment, which is more popularly known as the primary survey.

The contents of this survey can be remembered by using the mnemonic **DR ABC**.

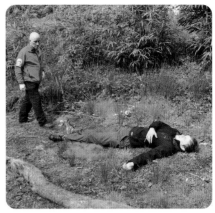

D Dangers

The first step in the primary survey is to check for dangers, which you would have already completed during the scene survey. It must be reiterated that your safety is the top priority and you should continue to be vigilant throughout the primary survey. Remember, failing to be alert to any further dangers could result in having more casualties to deal with, which could include yourself.

R Response

The next step is to check for a response to find out if the casualty is responsive or not. Approach the casualty, ideally from their feet (if space allows). This can reduce the risk of the casualty hyper-extending their neck should they be responsive.

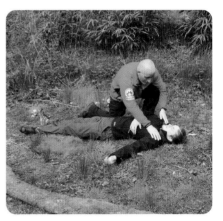

A RESPONSE CHECK CAN BE PERFORMED USING THE 'AVPU' SCALE:

Alert - If they are fully responsive, then ascertain the extent of their injury and deal with it appropriately.

Voice - "**Are you all right?**"
If they are not alert, then see if they will respond to a voice command.

Place your hands on their shoulders and gently shake them.
If they don't respond to a voice command, then try shaking them gently by the shoulders.
NB: do not shake them if you suspect a spinal or head injury.

Unresponsive -
If there is no response at all, they must be deemed as being unresponsive or unconscious.

If your casualty responds, leave them in the position in which you find them providing there's no further danger. Try to find out what is wrong with them and treat accordingly.

YOUR BYSTANDER

A bystander can be a great benefit to you such as:

- Calling the emergency services
- Managing bystanders and potential hazards
- Fetching the first aid kit and defibrillator if you have one available
- Consoling relatives, friends and other bystanders
- Helping you administer first aid if they are trained to do so
- Cleaning up the scene if necessary
- A support for you during the incident

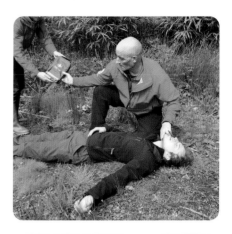

A Airway

Turn the casualty onto their back and then open the airway using the head tilt and chin lift method:

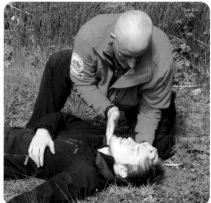

- Place your hand on their forehead and gently tilt their head back
- With two fingertips under the point of their chin, lift the chin to open the airway
- Be careful not to press on the fleshy part under the chin as it could restrict the airway

Support their head in this position in order to perform a breathing check.

Breathing

Look, listen and feel for normal breathing for no more than 10 seconds.

Look for chest movement

Listen at their mouth for breath sounds

Feel for air on your cheek

Support their head in the position shown below in order to perform a breathing check.

In the first few minutes after cardiac arrest, a casualty may be barely breathing, or taking infrequent, noisy, gasps. This is often termed agonal breathing or gasping, and must not be confused with normal breathing. If you have any doubt whether breathing is normal, act as if it is not normal and prepare to commence CPR.

Response to breathing check

The casualty who is unresponsive and not breathing normally is in cardiac arrest and requires CPR. Immediately following cardiac arrest blood flow to the brain is reduced to virtually zero, which may cause seizure-like episodes that may be confused with epilepsy. You should be suspicious of cardiac arrest with any casualty that presents seizure like symptoms and carefully assess whether they are breathing normally.

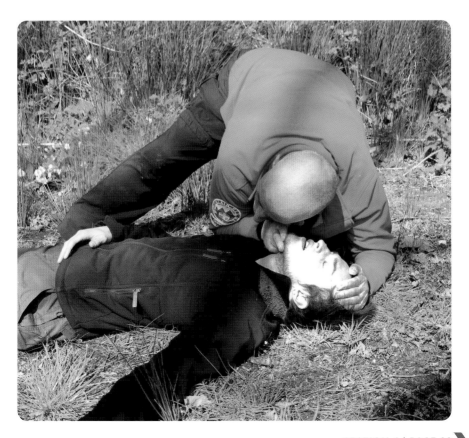

C CPR for a non-breathing casualty

Not breathing normally

If your casualty is not breathing normally, summon for professional medical assistance immediately. Lone rescuers should utilise the speaker function on their phone when making this call. If you have a bystander at hand, ask them to make this important call so that you can commence cardiopulmonary resuscitation (CPR) without delay.

You can also ask your bystander to unpack and prepare the Automated External Defibrillator (AED) if one is available. However, if you are on your own, then you will need to prepare the AED yourself, as quickly as possible.

Try and stay with your casualty when making the phone call if your signal permits. If you are able to, activate the speaker function on your phone to aid communication between you and the emergency services.

Breathing normally

If your casualty is breathing normally and has no major physical trauma, they should be placed in the recovery position.

If the casualty has physical trauma then the injuries should be treated accordingly and the casualty left in the position found.

However, if you believe their airway is at risk, then the recovery position should be used.

Ensure that you monitor the casualty's breathing whilst awaiting rescue.

If you are unsure about the extent of the injury, then you should perform a top-to-toe survey.

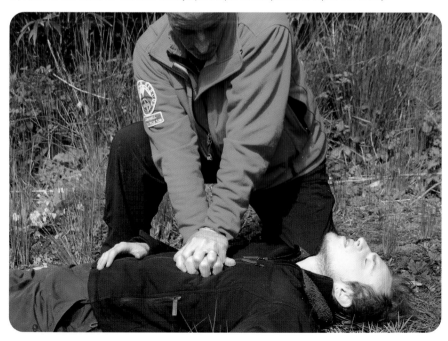

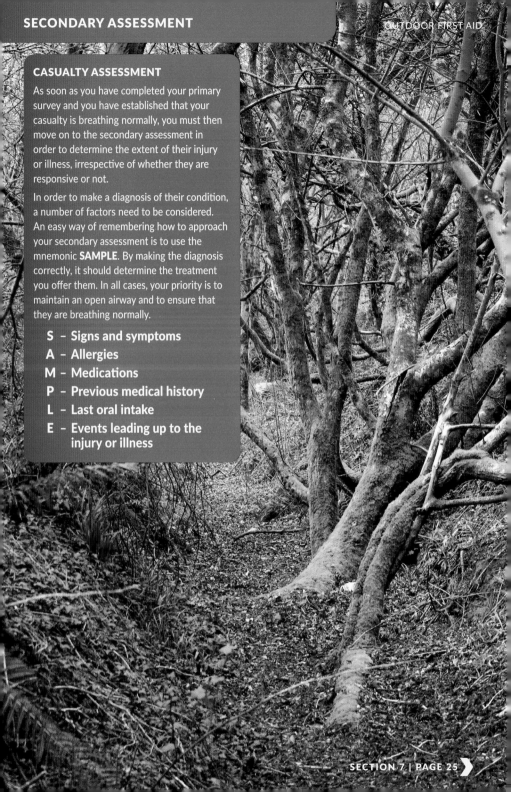

CASUALTY ASSESSMENT

As soon as you have completed your primary survey and you have established that your casualty is breathing normally, you must then move on to the secondary assessment in order to determine the extent of their injury or illness, irrespective of whether they are responsive or not.

In order to make a diagnosis of their condition, a number of factors need to be considered. An easy way of remembering how to approach your secondary assessment is to use the mnemonic **SAMPLE**. By making the diagnosis correctly, it should determine the treatment you offer them. In all cases, your priority is to maintain an open airway and to ensure that they are breathing normally.

S – **Signs and symptoms**
A – **Allergies**
M – **Medications**
P – **Previous medical history**
L – **Last oral intake**
E – **Events leading up to the injury or illness**

S – Signs and symptoms

What can you see in respect of the injury or condition? Use all your other senses. What can you smell, hear and feel? The casualty may be able to describe their symptoms to you.

A – Allergies

Ask your casualty if they suffer from any allergies. They may have suffered from an allergic reaction which has caused their condition, or they may be allergic to certain types of medication, or for instance latex (gloves), which could make their condition worse.

M – Medications

Ask your casualty about their condition. Do they have their own medication? Has it happened before? If they are currently taking prescription medication, make a note of the type, how often they take it and how much they take.

P – Previous medical history

Your casualty may have suffered from an injury or illness in the past which may account for their current condition. Ensure you make a note of any medical conditions your casualty has suffered from in the past so that you can make the emergency services aware when they arrive and take over from you.

L – Last oral intake

Ask your casualty when they last ate or drank. This is very important as their condition may have been caused by the food or drink they have consumed.

E – Events leading up to the injury or illness

If you were not present at the time of the incident, ask your casualty what they think may have happened leading up to the injury or illness.

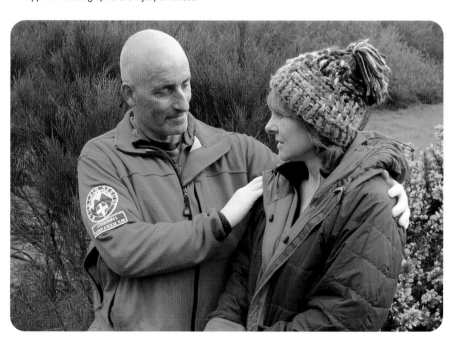

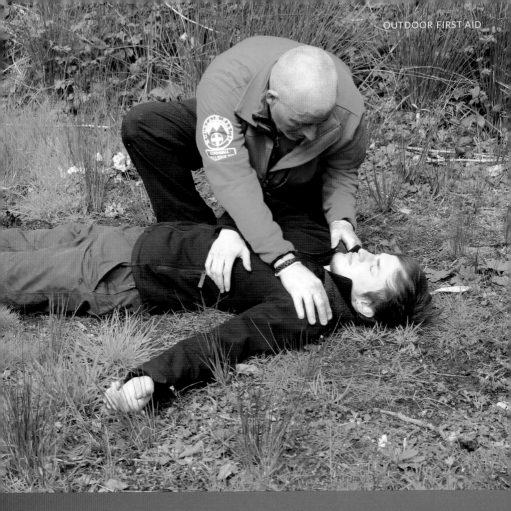

TOP-TO-TOE SURVEY

You will need to conduct a top-to-toe survey to examine the casualty's condition so that you can offer them the appropriate treatment. As the term suggests, you should start at their head and work your way down to their feet. You should wear gloves throughout this survey. Performing a top-to-toe survey in the outdoor environment may prove challenging due to possible space constraints, weather conditions and if the casualty is wearing thick layers of clothing.

Head, face and neck

Ensure that the airway is clear and that there are no visible obstructions. Look for bleeding, or any loss of fluids from the ears, eyes, nose and mouth. Feel for bumps, indentations and swelling around the head. Smell for unusual odour on the breath. Look for abnormal skin colouring and check the surface temperature.

Chest and shoulders

Check the collarbones for any fracture or deformity. Check the casualty's face for a response if you do suspect anything abnormal whilst assessing. Again, gently squeeze the rib-cage for anything abnormal and check for a response. Look at the rise and fall of the chest for abnormal breathing.

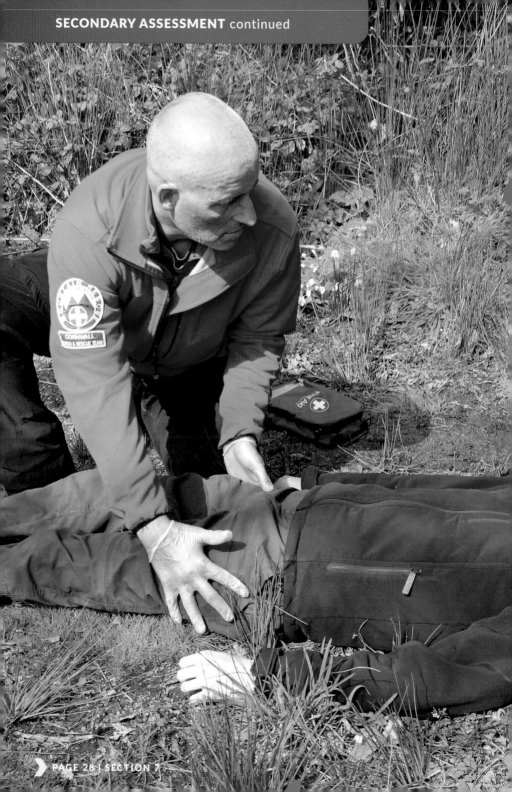

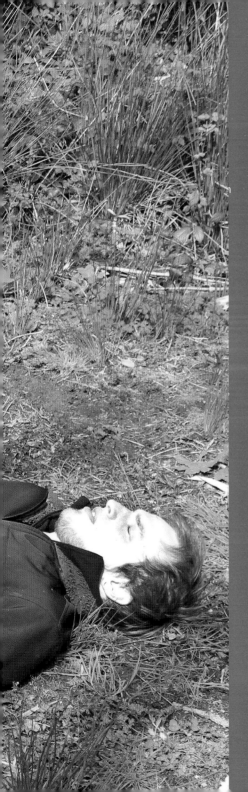

Arms

Check each arm for obvious signs of trauma including blood loss and swelling. Check for needle marks. See if the casualty is wearing an identity bracelet that may tell you of any condition they may have such as diabetes, anaphylaxis etc. Check the hands for bruising and disfigurement. Check for needle marks between the fingers.

Legs and extremities

Check each leg and foot for obvious signs of trauma including blood loss and swelling. If you suspect a fracture, then it is imperative that you immobilise the limb and prevent any movement.

Check the ankles for bruising and possible needle marks. When you have completed this survey, now is the time to call the emergency services ensuring that they are aware of any injury, as well the extent of it.

Your priority as a First Aider is to maintain an open airway for your casualty. If the casualty has no major physical trauma, you must place them in the recovery position and monitor them whilst waiting for the emergency services to arrive.

If the airway is compromised in any way then, irrespective of the injury, the casualty must be placed in the recovery position.

You must take extreme care, particularly if you suspect a spinal injury or a fracture.

RECOVERY POSITION (SAFE AIRWAY POSITION)

If your casualty is unresponsive, but breathing normally, with no evidence of major physical trauma then your priority is to ensure that their airway is not compromised in any way and that it remains open. Rather than leaving them on their back, or in a slumped position, then an effective way of achieving this is to place them in the recovery position, also known as the safe airway position.

Not only does the recovery position keep the airway open, but it also allows vomit to drain from the mouth and prevents them from rolling onto their back should you have to leave them.

Casualties in the outdoor environment should be insulated from the ground and should be placed injured side down if possible (as with a head or chest injury). Always position the casualty so their face is going down the hill. Shelter the casualty from environmental factors if necessary, such as:

- Temperature, both hot and cold
- Windy conditions which could interfere with breathing
  (Face away from the wind or obstruct the wind from hitting the casualty's face)
- Shade the casualty from strong sunlight but do not restrict the airway

If it is achievable, insulate the casualty from the ground before placing them in the recovery position and provide shelter.

1. Remove the casualty's glasses, if present
2. Kneel beside your casualty and make sure that both their legs are straight
3. Place the arm nearest to you out at a right angle to their body, elbow bent with the hand palm-up. Do not force the arm, let it fall naturally, but close to this position

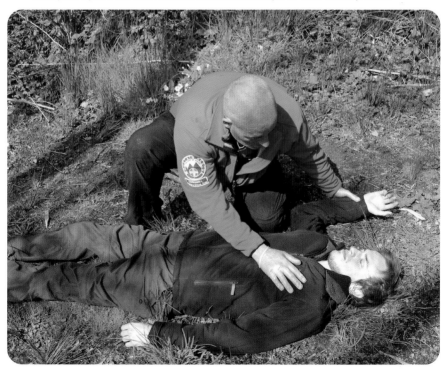

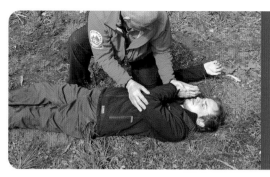

4. Bring the far arm across the chest, and hold the back of their hand against their cheek nearest to you

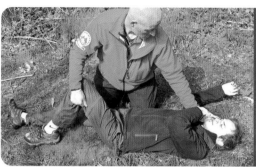

5. Grab hold of the far leg with your other hand, and raise the knee so that their foot is kept to the floor. This will be your lever for rolling them over

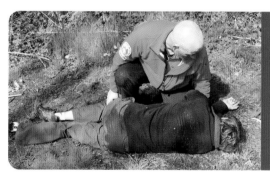

6. Keeping their hand pressed against their cheek, pull on the far leg to roll them towards you onto their side with their head supported all the way

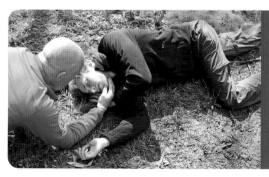

7. Tilt the head back to make sure that the airway remains open

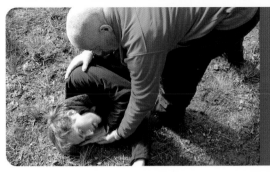

8. If necessary, adjust the hand under their cheek to keep the head tilted and facing downwards to allow liquid material to drain from the mouth

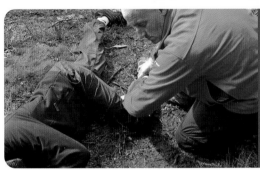

9. Adjust the upper leg so that both the hip and knee are bent at right angles

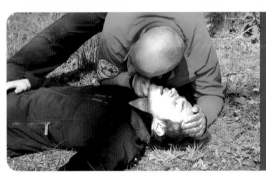

10. Check breathing regularly

11. If you have a bystander available to you, then this is the time to send them to call the emergency services, ensuring they have all the appropriate information and in particular, the condition of the casualty

12. If you have no bystander, you must call the emergency services yourself by dialling 999/112 and requesting the required service (Ambulance, Mountain Rescue etc)

If they have to be kept in the recovery position for more than 30 minutes, turn them to the opposite side to relieve the pressure on the lower arm. You must continue to monitor their breathing whilst waiting for professional medical help to take over. If they stop breathing normally, then you must call the emergency services with an update and commence CPR immediately.

It will also be worth monitoring other vital signs and noting other changes such as colouration of the skin, their temperature and responsiveness levels.

Pregnant women

Always put an unresponsive pregnant woman in the recovery position on her left side. This prevents compression of the inferior vena cava (large vein) by the uterus, which could be fatal for both the mother and the child.

Suspected spinal injury

If you suspect a spinal injury and you cannot maintain an open airway in the position you found them, care must be taken in moving them. Keep the casualty's back straight and support the head throughout. It would be extremely useful to have help in moving the casualty. The trained person should assume control when moving them.

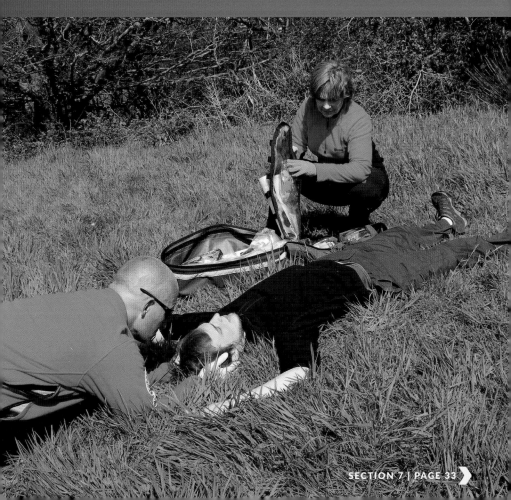

PRINCIPLES OF RESUSCITATION

Cardiopulmonary resuscitation (CPR) is an emergency procedure which is attempted in an effort to return life to a person who is not breathing normally for themselves.

This procedure combines chest compressions with rescue breaths. The chest compression replaces the heart's ability to pump oxygenated blood around the body, particularly to the vital organs such as the brain.

Rescue breathing provides the casualty, who is unable to breathe normally for themselves, valuable oxygen that is transported around the body by the chest compressions.

Without oxygen, brain damage can occur within three minutes. Therefore, your immediate action is paramount.

Referring back to Primary Survey, i.e. DR ABC, then you will have established that your casualty is not breathing normally.

Your immediate action now is to contact the emergency services, ensuring that you state that your casualty is not breathing normally.

If you have a bystander at hand, then send them to make this important call. You can also ask your bystander to unpack the Automated External Defibrillator (AED) and get it prepared for you, if one is available.

However, if you are on your own, then you must call the emergency services yourself. Stay with the casualty when making this call if possible.

If you are able to, activate the speaker function on your phone to aid communication between you and the emergency services.

Commence CPR without delay.

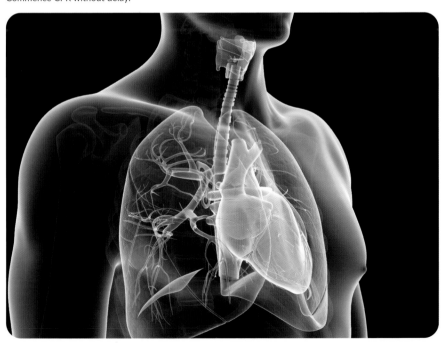

RESUSCITATION PROCEDURE

1. Start with 30 chest compressions

- **Kneel by the side of your casualty**
- **Place the heel of one hand in the centre of the casualty's chest - which is the lower half of the casualty's breastbone** (sternum)
- **Place the heel of your other hand on top of the first hand**
- **Interlock the fingers of your hands and ensure that pressure is not applied over their ribs. Do not apply any pressure over the upper abdomen or the bottom end of the sternum**
- **Position yourself vertically above their chest and, with your arms straight, press down on the sternum approximately 5cm** (But not more than 6cm)
- **After each compression, release all the pressure on the chest without losing contact between your hands and the sternum. Do not lean on the chest**
- **Repeat 30 chest compressions at a speed of 100 - 120 compressions per minute with as few interruptions as possible**
- **Compression and release should take an equal amount of time**

In most circumstances, it will be possible to identify the correct hand position for chest compressions, without removing the casualty's clothes. If you are in any doubt, then remove outer clothing.

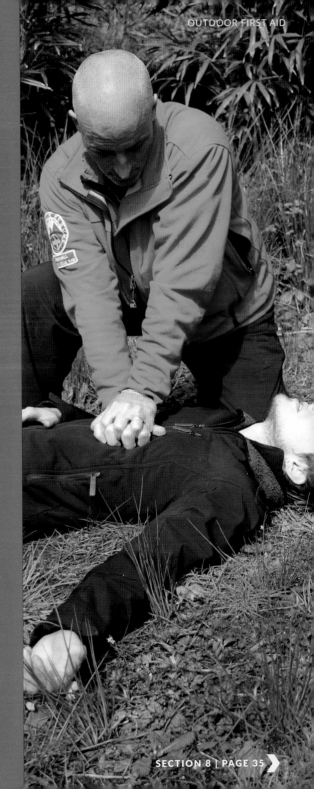

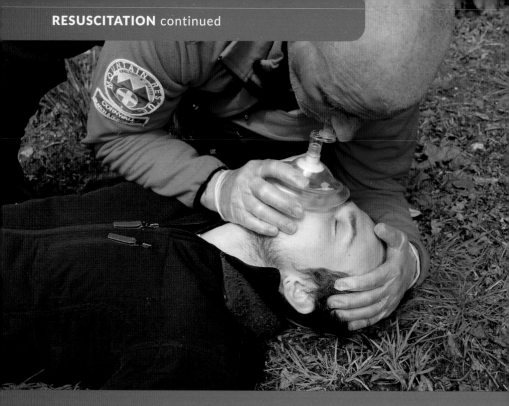

2. GIVE 2 RESCUE BREATHS

After 30 chest compressions open the airway again using head tilt and chin lift.

- Pinch the soft part of their nose closed, using the index finger and thumb of your hand on their forehead
- Allow their mouth to open, but maintain chin lift
- Take a normal breath and place your lips around their mouth, making sure that you have a good seal
- Blow steadily into their mouth whilst watching for their chest to rise, taking about one second as in normal breathing; this is an effective rescue breath
- Maintaining head tilt and chin lift, watch for their chest to fall as air comes out
- Take another normal breath and blow into the casualty's mouth once more to achieve a total of two effective rescue breaths. Do not interrupt compressions by more than 10 seconds to deliver two breaths. Then return your hands without delay to the correct position on the sternum and give a further 30 chest compressions

If the initial rescue breath of each sequence does not make the chest rise as in normal breathing, then, before your next attempt:

- Check the casualty's mouth and remove any visible obstruction
- Re-check that there is adequate head tilt and chin lift
- Do not attempt more than two breaths each time before returning to chest compressions

REPEAT 30 COMPRESSIONS AND 2 BREATHS UNTIL:

- **A health professional tells you to stop**
- **The casualty is definitely waking up, moving, opening their eyes and breathing normally**
- **You become exhausted**

It is rare for CPR alone to restart the heart. Unless you are certain the casualty has recovered, continue with CPR. Signs the casualty has recovered include:

- **Waking up**
- **Moving**
- **Opens eyes**

  and/or

- **They start breathing normally again**

Be prepared to **restart CPR immediately** if the casualty deteriorates.

It must be emphasised that if you are unable to give rescue breaths for whatever reason, then you must continue with **chest-compression-only CPR**. If there is more than one rescuer present, another should take over CPR about every 1-2 minutes to prevent fatigue. Ensure the minimum of delay during the changeover of rescuers and do not interrupt chest compressions.

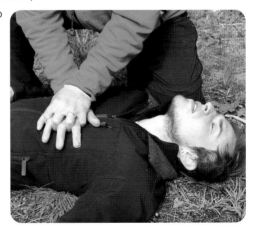

If you have access to an AED

As soon as it arrives, switch it on and attach the electrode pads on the casualty's chest. Follow the voice prompts. If more than one rescuer is present, CPR should be continued whilst the electrode pads are being attached to the chest.

NB: If your casualty is in a wet environment, such as a riverbank, move them to a dry area before applying the AED electrode pads.

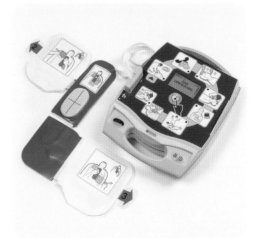

THE CHAIN OF SURVIVAL

It is critical that you follow this chain when you are dealing with a casualty who is not breathing normally.

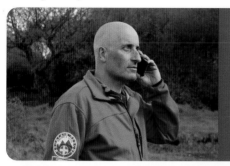

Early recognition and call for help

Call or send for help and fetch the defibrillator if you have one available. **Dial 999/112** to summon for professional medical assistance.

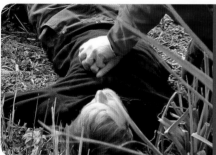

Early CPR

Start CPR to buy time until medical help arrives.

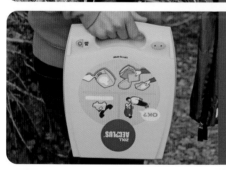

Early defibrillation

Defibrillators give an electric shock to re-organise the rhythm of the heart. Defibrillation within 3–5 minutes of cardiac arrest can produce survival rates as high as 50–70%. Each minute of delay to defibrillation reduces the probability of survival to hospital discharge by 10%.

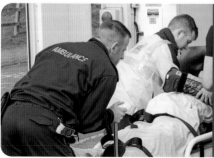

Post-resuscitation care

Professional help in order to restore the quality of life. Casualty needs to be transferred to a hospital immediately.

ADULT BASIC LIFE SUPPORT ALGORYTHYM

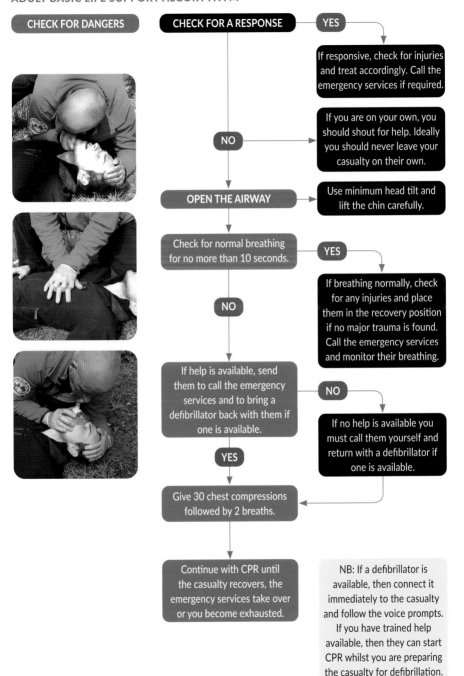

CHECK FOR DANGERS

CHECK FOR A RESPONSE

YES

If responsive, check for injuries and treat accordingly. Call the emergency services if required.

NO

If you are on your own, you should shout for help. Ideally you should never leave your casualty on their own.

OPEN THE AIRWAY

Use minimum head tilt and lift the chin carefully.

Check for normal breathing for no more than 10 seconds.

YES

If breathing normally, check for any injuries and place them in the recovery position if no major trauma is found. Call the emergency services and monitor their breathing.

NO

If help is available, send them to call the emergency services and to bring a defibrillator back with them if one is available.

NO

If no help is available you must call them yourself and return with a defibrillator if one is available.

YES

Give 30 chest compressions followed by 2 breaths.

Continue with CPR until the casualty recovers, the emergency services take over or you become exhausted.

NB: If a defibrillator is available, then connect it immediately to the casualty and follow the voice prompts. If you have trained help available, then they can start CPR whilst you are preparing the casualty for defibrillation.

DROWNING

Drowning is defined as respiratory impairment from being in, or under a liquid, normally water.

Drowning begins as a result of the casualty not being able to breathe because the airways are submerged below the surface of the liquid.

As with any incident, follow the Primary Survey protocol:

DANGERS

Consider the risk to yourself before attempting to rescue the casualty.

It may well be that chemicals are involved causing an additional toxic risk e.g. a slurry tank.

RESPONSE

Check for a response as you would normally do.

AIRWAY

Open the airway

BREATHING

Check to see if they are breathing normally.

CPR

If they are not breathing normally, shout for help and call 999 unless you have help at hand and then send them to make the call and to find an AED.

CPR PROCEDURE

- Call 999
- Open the airway
- Give 5 initial rescue breaths
- Follow with 30 chest compressions
- Repeat 2 rescue breaths followed by 30 chest compressions until the casualty recovers, or the emergency services take over from you
- Attach the AED when it arrives and follow the voice prompts. Ensure there is no direct contact with the casualty and the water when defibrillating

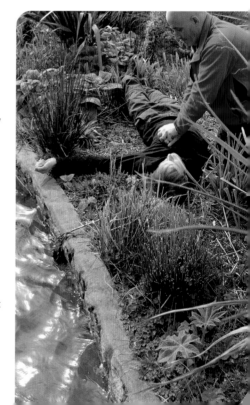

Many casualties that drown will regurgitate their stomach contents. If this is the case, roll them on to their side so that it drains out leaving a clear and open airway.

If the casualty recovers, put them into the recovery position, keep them warm and continue to monitor them.

If they are not breathing normally, shout for help and call the emergency services. If you have help at hand, send them to make this important call.

OTHER METHODS OF RESUSCITATION

Mouth to nose

This is where you seal off your casualty's mouth by pressing the chin upwards and breathe directly into the casualty's nose.

- **With your casualty's head tilted back, close the mouth by pushing up on their chin**
- **Seal your mouth around your casualty's nose and deliver a rescue breath**
- **After delivering the rescue breath, open your casualty's mouth to let out air**
- **Deliver the second breath and then continue with CPR (30:2)**

This method may be used if you suspect your casualty has ingested some form of poison, or where there is trauma to the mouth area.

Mouth to neck breather (stoma)

This method is used for a casualty who has an airway device or artificial opening in their throat. This opening is known as a 'stoma'.

- **Check your casualty's neck to see if they breathe through a stoma**
- **You will need to create a tight seal around the stoma, or use a pocket mask to create the seal**
- **Deliver the rescue breath into the stoma whilst holding your casualty's mouth closed**
- **If your rescue breath is successful, their chest should rise and fall and you should be able to feel and hear the air escaping from the stoma**
- **Deliver the second breath and then continue with CPR (30:2)**

Face shields and pocket masks

In order to reduce the risk of cross-contamination, there are various protective shields and masks available that will significantly reduce this risk.

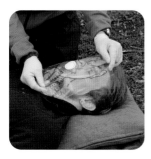 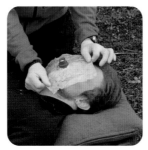 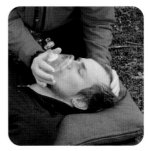

PAEDIATRIC RESUSCITATION

The term paediatric refers to children and infants (babies). A child is deemed as being aged from 1-18 years old and an infant or baby, being aged under 1 year old.

CPR FOR AN INFANT

CPR FOR A CHILD

IF YOU HAVE HELP AVAILABLE
Ask them to call the emergency services immediately.

The following modifications to the adult sequence will make it more suitable for use in infants:

- Carefully remove any obvious airway obstructions
- Give 5 initial rescue breaths

Take a breath and cover the mouth and nose of the infant with your mouth, making sure you have a good seal. If both the nose and mouth cannot be covered in the older infant, then attempt to seal only the infant's nose or mouth with your mouth (if the nose is used, close the lips to prevent air escape and vice versa). Blow steadily until the chest rises.

The following modifications to the adult sequence will make it more suitable for use in children:

- Carefully remove any obvious airway obstructions
- Give 5 initial rescue breaths

Pinch the soft part of their nose closed with the index finger and thumb of your hand on their forehead. Take a normal breath and form a good seal around the child's mouth with your mouth. Blow steadily until the chest rises.

IF YOU ARE ON YOUR OWN
Perform CPR for 1 minute i.e. approximately 2 cycles of 30 chest compressions followed by 2 rescue breaths. You must then call 999/112 yourself.

TECHNIQUE FOR GIVING CHEST COMPRESSIONS FOR AN INFANT

- Compress the chest by at least one-third of its depth which is approximately 4cm for an infant
- Use the tips of 2 fingers to compress the chest
- The compression rate should be between 100–120 per minute

TECHNIQUE FOR GIVING CHEST COMPRESSIONS FOR A CHILD

- Compress the chest by at least one-third of its depth which is approximately 5cm for a child
- Use one or two hands for a child over 1 year to achieve an adequate depth of compression
- The compression rate should be between 100–120 per minute

Continue with CPR (30:2) until the emergency services take over from you, your casualty recovers* or you become too exhausted to continue.

Should an AED arrive, unpack it and connect it to your casualty. Follow the voice prompts.

*Recovery means that they start to show signs of life i.e. they wake up, or start moving, or open their eyes **and** they start to breathe normally for themselves.

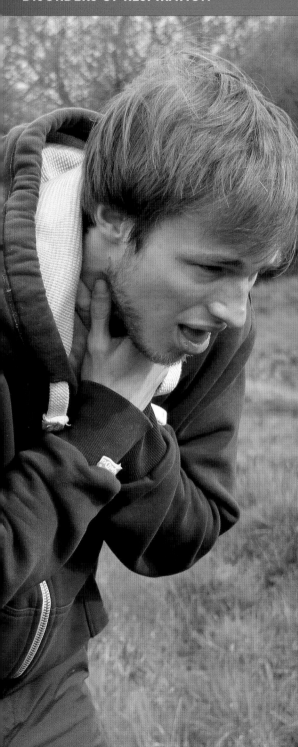

CHOKING

There are many factors that can contribute to a respiratory disorder, including asthma, hypoxia, smoke inhalation and choking. Choking is probably the most common of the disorders and probably the most distressing to suffer and to deal with. Your immediate treatment is required.

Should your casualty become unresponsive as a result of choking, then you will have to start resuscitation.

You should suspect choking if someone is unable to speak or talk, particularly if they're eating.

Recognition of someone choking

- **Difficulty in speaking and breathing**
- **Coughing or gagging**
- **Clutching at the throat and pointing to the mouth**
- **Pale, grey/blue skin tone in the later stages** (cyanosis)
- **Ultimately – unresponsiveness**

If your casualty shows signs of a mild or partial airway obstruction then:

- **Encourage them to cough**
- **Stay calm and offer plenty of encouragement and reassurance**

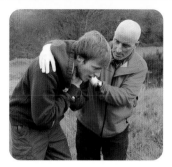

If coughing becomes ineffective, then provide treatment for a severe airway obstruction for an adult:

- Check their mouth and remove any obvious obstruction

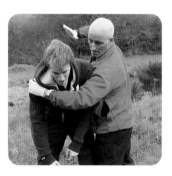

Bend them forward and give up to five back blows.

- Stand to the side and slightly behind your casualty
- Support the chest with one hand and lean them forward so that when the obstruction is dislodged it comes out of the mouth rather than to go further down the airway
- Give up to five sharp blows between their shoulder blades with the heel of your other hand
- Check to see if each back blow has relieved the airway obstruction. The aim is to relieve the obstruction with each blow rather than to give all five unnecessarily

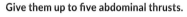

Give them up to five abdominal thrusts.

- Stand behind your casualty and put both arms round the upper part of their abdomen
- Lean them forward
- Clench your fist and place it between the umbilicus (navel) and the bottom end of their sternum (breastbone)
- Grasp this hand with your other hand and pull sharply inwards and upwards
- Repeat up to five times
- Check to see if each abdominal thrust has relieved the airway obstruction. The aim is to relieve the obstruction with each thrust rather than to give all five unnecessarily

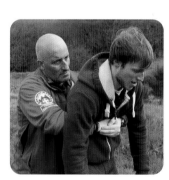

If you have performed abdominal thrusts on your casualty, they must be sent to hospital to be examined for any internal injuries.

If the obstruction cannot be removed after the first cycle of back blows and abdominal thrusts, then you must call the emergency services immediately. Repeat the process of up to five back blows followed by up to five abdominal thrusts until the casualty recovers, or professional medical help arrives and take over from you.

If your casualty becomes unresponsive, then help them to the floor onto their back. **Dial 999/112**, and commence CPR immediately. Before each rescue breath attempt, check in the mouth for any visible obstruction that can be removed easily without having to sweep the mouth with your fingers.

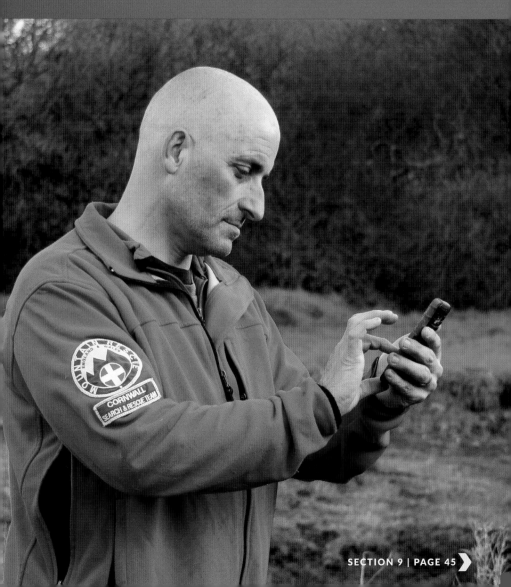

THE CIRCULATORY SYSTEM

The circulatory system is our body's transport system for two fluids, namely, blood and lymph.

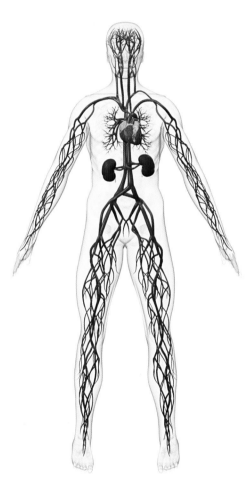

For the purposes of first aid the focus is on the transport of blood, also known as the cardio-vascular system.

This system consists of the heart and blood vessels, which supply our body, and in particular, our vital organs such as the brain and heart, with blood containing oxygen and nutrients to keep them healthy.

Our heart is a hollow muscular pump, about the size of your fist, with two pairs of chambers. These chambers collect blood flowing back from our body after depositing the oxygen and nutrients, before being pumped back to the lungs to collect more oxygen so that the cycle of transportation can continue.

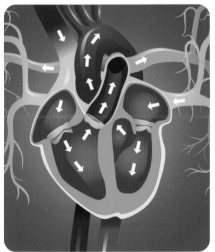

The adult heart beats approximately 60 – 80 times every minute and pumps approximately six litres of blood around our body every minute.

Blood is carried around the body by vessels known as arteries, veins and capillaries.

When a blood vessel is torn or severed, blood loss and shock cause the blood pressure to fall and the injured vessels will contract at the injury site.

Platelets and proteins come into contact with the injured site and 'plug' the wound. This process begins within ten minutes if the loss of blood is brought under control.

BLOOD COMPOSITION

The blood vessels within this system are:

- **Arteries**

  Deliver oxygenated blood from the heart to the body, with the exception of the pulmonary artery which carries de-oxygenated blood from the heart to the lungs.

- **Veins**

  Carry the de-oxygenated blood back to the heart.

- **Capillaries**

Much smaller vessels that form a link between the arteries, veins and body tissue to allow the transfer of oxygen and nutrients to the body and the waste products to be removed.

Blood is made up of:

- **Plasma**

  The fluid component of the blood of which 90% is water.

- **Platelets**

  Help to block the blood flow by clotting.

- **Red cells**

  Transport the oxygen via the haemoglobin.

- **White cells**

  Manufacture antibodies and fight infection and bacteria.

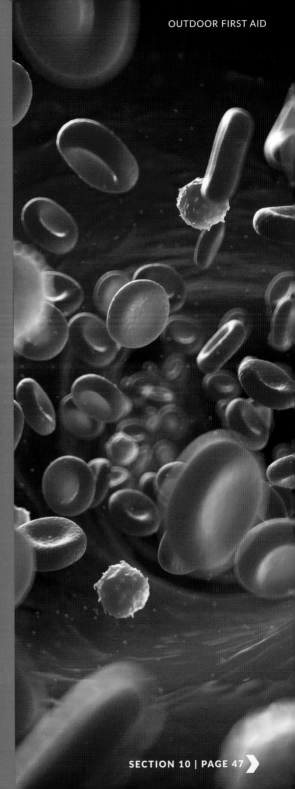

TYPES OF WOUND

A wound can be best described as a type of injury in which the skin is torn, cut or punctured (an open wound), or where a blunt force created a contusion (a bruise).

In first aid, there are 6 types of wounds that you should be familiar with:

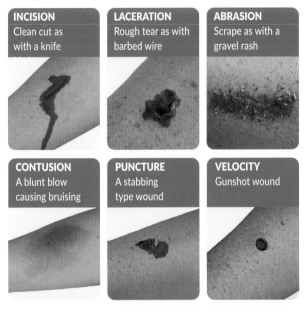

INCISION
Clean cut as with a knife blade

LACERATION
Rough tear as with barbed wire

ABRASION
Scrape as with a gravel rash

CONTUSION
A blunt blow causing bruising

PUNCTURE
A stabbing type wound

VELOCITY
Gunshot wound

TYPES OF BLEEDING

Bleeding is classified by the type of blood vessel that is damaged.

Arterial Pumps from the wound with the heartbeat

Venous Gushes from the wound or pools at the site

Capillary Oozing at the site of injury

Once you have completed your initial casualty assessment for prioritising your treatment, you must follow the guidelines for personal protection and hygiene control before you begin to treat the casualty for bleeding.

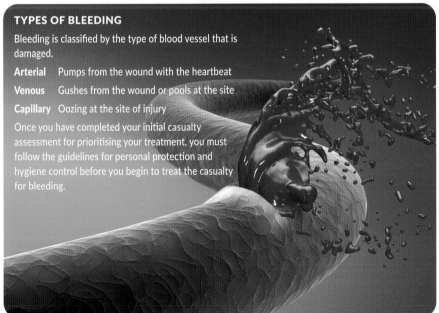

TREATMENT FOR THE CONTROL OF BLEEDING

- **Wear disposable gloves**
- **Expose and examine the wound**
- **Apply direct pressure with your fingers or palm, preferably over a sterile dressing or non-fluffy clean pad** (you can ask your casualty to apply this pressure)
- **Elevate and support an injured limb for cuts that are NOT catastrophic**
- **Help the casualty to lie down and raise the legs if you suspect shock**

Cleaning wounds

If you have first aid cleaning supplies available, you should clean the wound to reduce the risk of infection, before applying a sterile dressing.

In an ideal situation, you will have running water available from a mains supply. If you are in a remote setting where running water is not available, you can use bottled drinking water, saline solution (salt water solution) or alcohol-free wipes to clean the wound.

- **Secure the dressing with a bandage large enough to cover the wound**
- **If blood seeps through this dressing, remove both the dressing and bandage and apply pressure to the bleed with a new dressing**
- **Secure the new dressing with a bandage once the bleeding is under control**
- **Support the injured limb with a sling or bandaging if appropriate, providing the casualty allows you to do so**
- **Monitor vital signs and summon the emergency services if necessary**

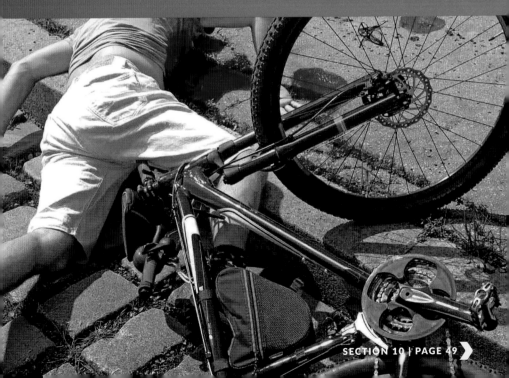

CATASTROPHIC BLEEDING

If you are unable to stop the bleeding due to the severity of the injury, you will need to apply direct pressure continually and then pack the wound with haemostatic dressings, or apply a tourniquet.

If you have neither, then you must continue to apply direct pressure and consider making an improvised tourniquet. It is imperative that you call for professional medical help immediately for a severe, or catastrophic bleed.

To summarise the treatment for catastrophic bleeding:

- **Do apply direct pressure to the wound**
- **Do use a haemostatic dressing or tourniquet**
- **Do not apply indirect pressure to proximal pressure points**
- **Do not elevate an extremity**

HAEMOSTATIC DRESSINGS

A haemostatic dressing is a medical dressing used to control blood loss by accelerating the clotting process. The dressing is impregnated with a special agent that when it makes contact with a fluid (blood in this instance), it creates a gel around the point of where the blood is being lost, which in essence, acts as the clot, or 'pseudo' clot. This special agent also comes in a granular and powder form.

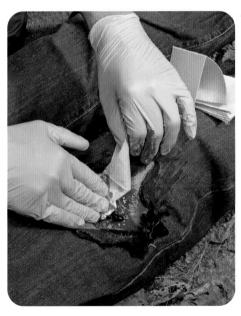

Haemostatic dressings are commonly used to control bleeding in surgical and military settings, especially when the wound is an area such as the neck, abdomen or groin where compression is not possible.

It would prove useful to pack haemostatic dressings in your first aid container before entering a remote setting as the relevant emergency service may take a considerable amount of time to reach you and controlling a catastrophic bleed with direct pressure alone may not be possible.

General points to remember:

- Always apply direct pressure to the wound first, before applying a haemostatic dressing or haemostatic agent
- Training must be given on how to apply this type of dressing or agent
- Send the packaging with the casualty to the hospital so that they know what has been applied
- Check the expiry date on the packaging
- Do not use a haemostatic agent on an open chest wound, open head injury, the airway or the eyes

For a catastrophic bleed, the priorities of the Primary Survey would change to:

D   Check for dangers

R   Response

C   Catastrophic bleed identified
This is now your priority. Summon for professional medical help immediately and control the bleeding.

A   Airway

B   Breathing

C   CPR/Circulation

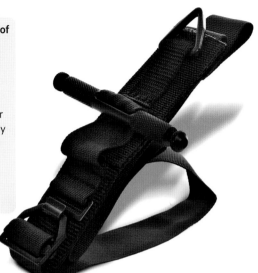

TOURNIQUETS

A tourniquet is a band that's wrapped tightly around a limb to stop blood loss. Tourniquets have been used in military settings for severe external limb bleeding for many years. A tourniquet should be used when direct wound pressure cannot control severe external bleeding in a limb.

General points to remember:

- A windlass is part of a tourniquet that is twisted to tighten it and is then locked or tied in place to secure the tourniquet when pressure is applied
- A tourniquet should be a minimum of 1.5 inches wide and this is particularly important if you have to improvise and make your own
- Unpack the manufactured tourniquet and have it ready for use
- Apply directly to the skin and not clothing
- Make sure you write the time of application on the tourniquet. Most manufactured ones will have an area dedicated to this

A tourniquet should only be used as a last resort with external bleeding that could have life threatening consequences, or an amputation. Therefore, you must do all you can to prevent the condition from worsening especially in the remote environment where rescue or medical assistance may be some time away.

> It must be emphasised that further training is required for First Aiders in respect of using haemostatic dressings or tourniquets.
>
> Please speak to your training provider.

EMBEDDED OBJECTS

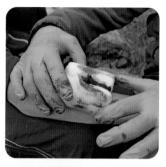

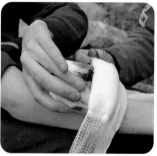

If during your examination of the wound you see an embedded object such as a shard of rock or piece of glass, then you must leave it in place and dress around it. Your aim is to stop the bleeding, but care must be taken not to put any direct pressure on the embedded object.

1 Check the wound for anything embedded

2 Do not attempt to remove or move the object

3 Apply dressing and pressure to either side of the object

4 Apply a larger sterile dressing over the top

5 Secure the bandage

6 Insulate the casualty from the ground, provide shelter and elevate the injured limb

7 Treat for shock

8 Summon for professional medical help by dialling 999/112

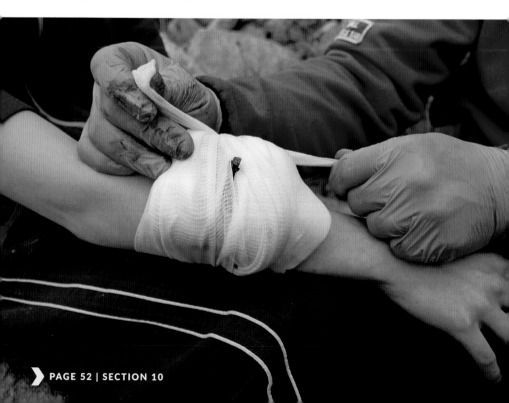

BLEEDING FROM ORIFICES

Signs, symptoms and causes

Site	Appearance	Cause
Mouth	Bright red, frothy, coughed up. Vomited blood, red or dark reddish brown.	Bleeding in the lungs. Bleeding in the stomach.
Ear	Fresh bright-red blood. Thin, watery blood.	Injury to ear, perforated eardrum. Head injury.
Nose	Fresh bright red blood. Thin, watery blood.	Ruptured blood vessel in nostril. Skull fracture.
Anus	Fresh bright-red blood. Black tarry, offensive smelling stool.	Injury to anus or lower bowel. Injury to upper bowel.
Urethra	Urine with red or smoky appearance and occasional clots.	Bleeding from the bladder, kidneys.
Vagina	Either fresh or dark blood	Menstruation, miscarriage, disease or injury to the vagina or womb.

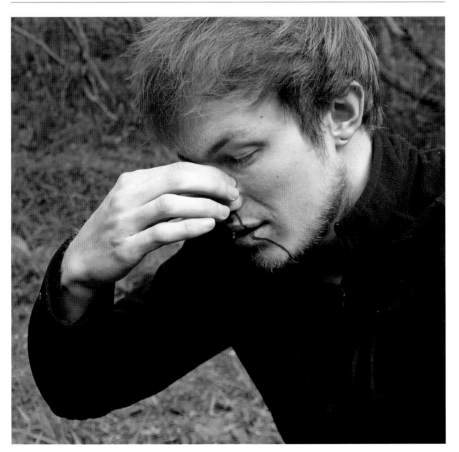

BLEEDING FROM ORIFICES – TREATMENT

- Treat the cause where possible using sterile dressings
- Treat your casualty for shock
- Monitor their condition, particularly their breathing
- Call the emergency services
- Insulate the casualty from the ground, provide shelter and monitor vital signs
- Lay them injured side down where possible
- Do not try to plug the wound, but cover it with a sterile dressing
- Offer them plenty of reassurance
- Pay attention to the casualty's modesty and dignity, particularly if they are bleeding from the anus or vagina

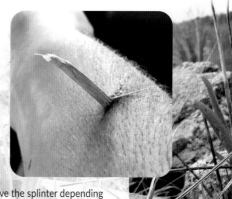

SPLINTERS

A splinter is a fragment of a larger object that penetrates into the skin causing pain and discomfort. Splinters in the outdoor environment could be caused by vegetative materials such as pine needles and thorns. Plastic, glass and metal fragments can also pierce into the skin causing problems.

You will need to decide if it is appropriate to remove the splinter depending on the size of the fragment, the depth of the wound and the type of material embedded.

Treatment

- Wear disposable gloves
- Clean the area around the splinter
- Grip the splinter with tweezers as close to the skin as possible
- Carefully pull the splinter out in a straight line, following the same angle as it went into the skin
- Once removed, thoroughly clean the wound
- Cover with a sterile dressing

If the splinter is fully embedded, cover with a sterile dressing and seek medical attention.

AMPUTATIONS

Any part of the body that has been severed will need immediate hospital treatment. There is almost certain to be severe blood loss, and your aim as a First Aider is to control the bleeding, treat for shock and to protect and transport the amputated body part to hospital with the casualty.

Your prompt and effective treatment may just allow the amputated part to be stitched back successfully with micro-surgery.

Signs and symptoms

- Bleeding
- Shock
- Severe pain in the majority of cases
- An open wound
- Amputated body part

Treatment

- Ensure that the area is safe for you and your casualty
- Reduce the risk of cross-infection by wearing disposable gloves
- Control the loss of blood by applying direct pressure with a sterile, non-fluffy dressing
- Treat your casualty for shock
- Call the emergency services
- Wrap the amputated part in plastic such as cling-film
- Wrap it further in a cloth
- Submerge the wrapped and protected part in ice or snow if available. Otherwise, instant ice packs can be used where you 'break' the packet to activate the 'ice' mixture. It is important that the severed part does not make direct contact with the ice
- Mark the package clearly with your casualty's name and ensure that it is transported to hospital with your casualty
- Insulate your casualty from the ground, provide shelter and monitor vital signs whilst awaiting rescue
- Protect and maintain an open airway
- Be prepared to resuscitate if your casualty stops breathing normally

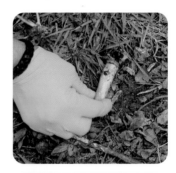

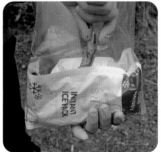

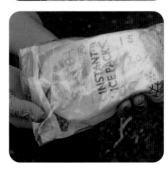

MINOR CUTS AND GRAZES

Cuts and grazes are some of the most common outdoor injuries. Minor cuts and grazes (where only the surface layer of skin is cut or scraped off) may bleed and feel slightly painful, but the affected area will normally scab over and heal quickly.

However, if the cut is in an area that is constantly moving, such as your knee joint, it may take longer to heal.

Depending on how deep the cut is and where it is on your body, a scar may remain once the cut has healed.

Deeper cuts may damage important structures below the skin such as nerves, blood vessels or tendons.

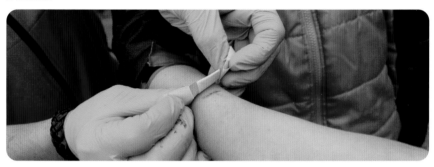

Most cuts and grazes can be easily treated by cleaning them thoroughly and covering them with a plaster or dressing.

Seek medical help if any of the below apply:

You think there is damage to deeper tissues: signs include numbness (indicating injury to a nerve), blood spurting from the wound or bleeding that does not stop after five minutes of continuous firm pressure.

The wound is at risk of becoming infected: for example, a cut has been contaminated with soil, faeces or a dirty blade, or material such as grit and other debris which can be seen in the wound.

The wound has become infected: signs include swelling of the affected area, pus coming from the wound, redness spreading from the wound and increasing pain. The wound cannot be closed with a plaster, or it starts to open up when it moves.

The wound will create an unwelcome scar: for example, if it occurs on a prominent part of the casualty's face.

Tetanus immunisation

'Tetanus' is a serious but rare condition caused by bacteria usually from dirt and soil getting into an open wound on the body.

If your casualty's wound has been contaminated by dirt or soil, then it is advisable to ask your casualty about their history of tetanus immunisation. Advise to seek medical advice if:

- **They have never been immunised**
- **If they are unsure about their history of injections**

BRUISING

Bruises are bluish or purple-coloured patches that appear on the skin when tiny blood vessels (capillaries) break or burst underneath it.

The blood from the capillaries leak into the soft tissue under the skin causing the discolouration. Over time this fades through shades of yellow or green. Bruises often feel tender or swollen at first.

What causes bruising?

Bruising is caused by internal bleeding (under the skin) due to a person injuring themselves by, for example, falling over, walking into something or playing sports.

Some people are naturally more likely to bruise than others, for example, the elderly may bruise more easily because their skin is thinner and the tissue underneath is more fragile.

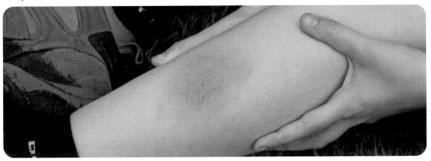

Treatment for bruises

Treat bruises, initially, by limiting the bleeding. You can do this by cooling the area with a cold compress (a flannel or cloth soaked in cold water) or an instant ice pack wrapped in a towel.

Hold the cold compress or similar over the affected area for at least 10 minutes.

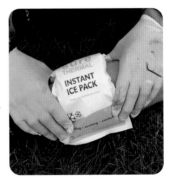

Do not put the instant ice pack straight onto the skin as this will possibly cause further damage. Most bruises will disappear after around two weeks.

If the bruise is still there after two weeks, you should recommend that your casualty see their GP.

Internal bruising

Bruises don't just happen under the skin - they can also happen deeper in the body's tissues, organs and bones.

While the bleeding isn't visible, the bruises can cause swelling and pain.

You should recommend that your casualty seeks medical attention, or summon for professional help if you feel the injury is of a serious nature, particularly if they have been involved in an accident such as a fall from height.

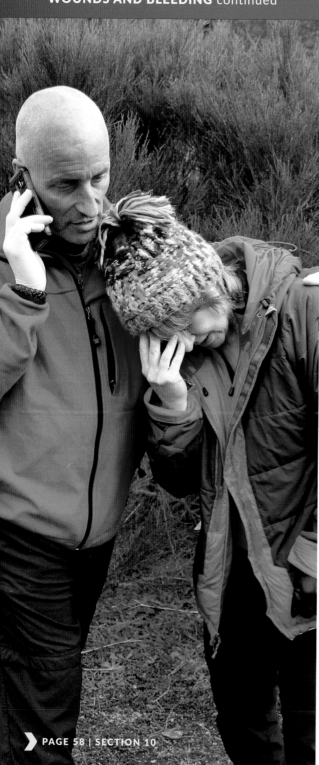

INTERNAL BLEEDING

Internal bleeding can occur after any physical injury and almost any organ or blood vessel can be affected by the trauma, which can lead to internal bleeding.

In the majority of cases, internal bleeding results from major injuries such as blunt trauma, penetrating trauma or severe crush injuries.

Sometimes internal bleeding can occur after less severe trauma. This can be very dangerous because the bleeding will continue and steadily get worse over time.

You will need to monitor their condition very closely and look out for symptoms such as:

- **Abdominal pain or swelling**
- **Unexplained chest pains**
- **Changes in skin colour**
- **External bleeding from an opening; Blood in stools, urine, vomit or vaginal bleeding**
- **External bruising**
- **Light headedness, dizziness or fainting**
- **Severe pain**
- **Weakness** (loss of strength)

If you are in any doubt regarding your casualty's condition, or if they are experiencing any of the above symptoms, seek professional medical assistance.

NOSEBLEEDS

A common injury that is caused generally by a direct blow or sneezing. However, high blood pressure can also cause a sudden bleed with little warning. If the blood is watery, then it could suggest a head injury, therefore making the incident far more serious i.e. possible skull fracture.

Treatment

- Insulate the ground, sit your casualty down and lean them forward
- Ask them to pinch the soft part of their nose as they lean forward
- Apply this pressure for 10 minutes and then release slowly
- Ask them to avoid rubbing or blowing their nose
- If you are unable to stop the bleeding, ask them to repeat the pinching process for a further 10 minutes

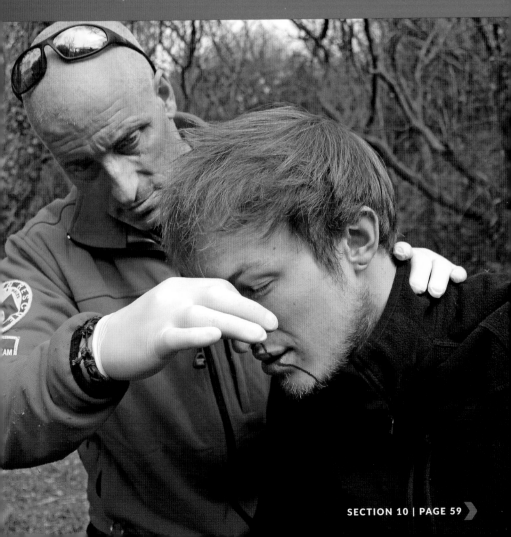

HYPOVOLAEMIC SHOCK

Hypovolaemic shock is best described as a failure or collapse of the circulatory system when the arterial blood pressure is too low to provide an adequate blood supply to the tissues.

There are a number of reasons why this system could fail, including blood loss, failure of the heart, poor circulation, a fall in blood pressure and the lack of oxygen contained within the body.

Other conditions include poisoning, vomiting, infection, burns and injury to the spinal cord, but this is by no means the definitive list.

As a First Aider, there are a number of things you can do for your casualty such as to stop the bleeding and to take pressure off the heart. One of your main concerns should be that hypovolaemic shock will set in very quickly if you don't react quickly enough, and shock can be a killer.

Signs and symptoms

- **Ashen coloured skin** (grey/blue)
- **Clammy and cold skin to touch**
- **Feeling of sickness and thirst**
- **Their breathing will be rapid and shallow**
- **Rapid, weak pulse**

Treatment

- **Deal with the injury or condition**
- **Make them comfortable by insulating from the ground, laying them down and providing shelter from the elements**
- **Raise both their legs providing it does not compromise their injuries further**
- **Keep them warm and maintain their response levels by talking to them**
- **Call the emergency services**
- **Monitor vital signs**
- **Do not allow them to smoke, eat or drink as it may affect their wellbeing and it could compromise further treatment**

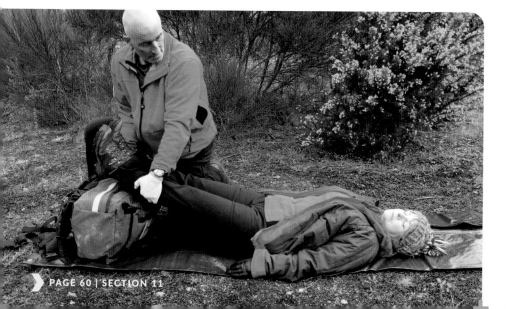

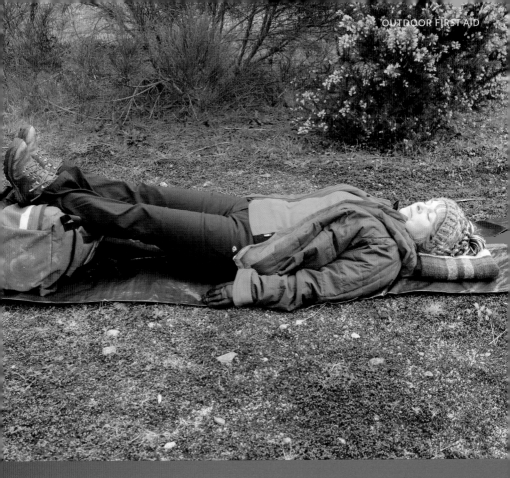

FAINTING

Fainting is a sudden, usually temporary, brief loss of responsiveness generally caused by insufficient oxygen in the brain. The signs and symptoms are the same as shock with the exception that the pulse rate is slower. A casualty who has fainted will generally make a rapid recovery and feel fine very quickly.

Treatment for someone who feels faint

- **Help them to the floor and lie them down**
- **Raise and support their legs**
- **Offer them plenty of fresh air**
- **Sit them up gradually**
- **Comfort and reassure them**

Treatment for someone who has fainted

If a person faints and does not regain responsiveness within one or two minutes, you should put them into the recovery position, monitor their breathing and call the emergency services as soon as possible.

MANAGING A CASUALTY IN OUTDOOR CLOTHING AND EQUIPMENT

When dealing with an incident that requires first aid, you may need to loosen, remove, open or even cut the casualty's clothing to provide effective treatment. The removal of clothing must be done in such a way that it does not make the injury or illness worse.

Ideally, you should treat your casualty under a group shelter, or tent if practicable. This will protect your casualty from the elements whilst you are treating them, reducing the risk of conditions such as hypothermia. Sheltering your casualty will also provide a form of privacy in the outdoor environment.

It will prove useful to pack a pair off tuff cut scissors which are perfect for cutting through thick clothing. If you need to cut your casualty's clothing to reach the injured area, be mindful of the scissor blades and try to lift away from your casualty when making the cut. If you need to repair the clothing after treatment, safety pins can be used as a temporary measure.

MOVING AND CARRYING A CASUALTY

There may be a time when you need to move your casualty to a safer position so that you can provide the necessary treatment, set-up shelter and make the job of applying first aid easier.

With non-critical injuries, it may be possible for your casualty to walk (with assistance) a short distance but it is important to weigh up the benefits and ask yourself, "will this make the situation better or worse?"

Fortunately, search and rescue teams can be called upon to assist with the emergency and provide all the necessary equipment to perform the evacuation, ranging from basic stretchers, to deploying a helicopter to assist with the rescue.

Immediately after an incident, professional medical help will not be available, so you may need to improvise and get your casualty to safety on your own, or with other members of your group. A good example of needing to move your casualty could be if they slipped on a bank and fell into a shallow river – this scenario certainly justifies moving and carrying your casualty, if it is safe for you to do so, as they are at risk of drowning and making their injuries worse.

Items of equipment used to move and carry your casualty may include:

- **Walking poles**
- **Rucksacks**
- **Climbing rope**
- **Group shelter**
- **Jackets/spare clothing**
- **Tarpaulin**
- **Emergency bivi bags**
- **Tent**

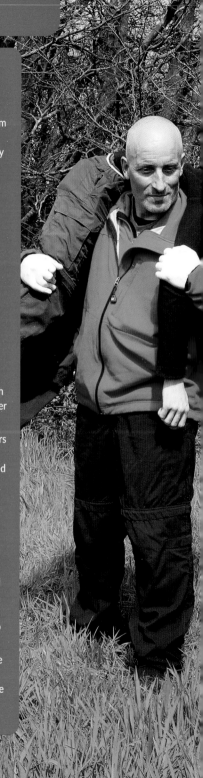

MOVING AND CARRYING A CASUALTY
WHEN YOU ARE ALONE

Walking with assistance

If your casualty is able to walk, you can physically assist them by offering your hand for support, or walking close by their side with their arm around your shoulders. Try and keep very close to the casualty in case they fall. If you have walking poles, they can be used for additional support and balance.

Firefighter's carry

A technique used in firefighting to carry casualties to safety away from a danger source. This can also be applied in outdoor first aid if you need to get away from a hazardous situation quickly.

The disadvantages of this type of carry is that it puts enormous strain on yourself, it can only really be used over short distances and it can be very uncomfortable for the casualty and possibly make their injuries worse.

Rucksack carry

A rucksack carry can be an effective method of carrying your casualty without any additional equipment. Place the rucksack on the floor and ask your casualty to step into each shoulder strap loop. Pull the rucksack up so that the shoulder straps are in their groin area.

Bend down and feed the rucksack straps onto your shoulders just as you would normally. Stand up slowly, bending your knees to avoid injury. Your casualty should now be supported on your back, just like a large rucksack.

Remember to continue talking to your casualty and offer plenty of reassurance, as it will be difficult to monitor any changes in vital signs when they are attached to your back.

One person rope carry

If you have a rope available, this can be used to carry your casualty over your back just like a rucksack. Make two equal coil sections from the rope and lay it on the floor (just like the figure 8). Ask your casualty to step into the loops, one foot in each section. Ask your casualty to pull the coils up to their groin.

Insert your arms into the upper section of the coil loops (one arm through each side), just like putting on a backpack. If your casualty is able to reach an elevated surface, this will be much easier for you when standing up as they will be at the same height.

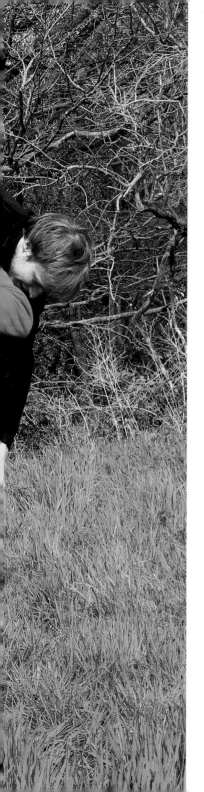

MOVING AND CARRYING A CASUALTY
WHEN YOU HAVE ASSISTANCE

Rucksack with walking poles carry

If you have a second person available and they are willing and able to help you move and carry the casualty, walking poles can be used as a seat between yours and the other persons rucksack.

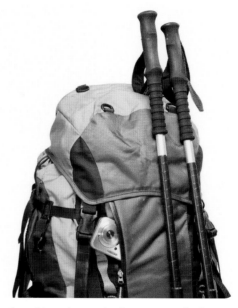

Tape the walking poles together for extra strength. Place the two rucksacks side by side on the ground and feed the taped walking poles through the gap near the bottom of the rucksacks, allowing enough space for the casualty to sit. Your casualty will need to be sat on top of the walking poles before you stand up slowly and cautiously, bending your knees to avoid injury. Ensure it is comfortable for your casualty as well as yourself. If in any doubt, stop and reassess the situation.

Two person rope carry

Similar to the one person rope carry, you will need to make two coil sections, but this time, you and the other person sling the coil loops over your shoulders, so that the middle knot acts as a seat for your casualty. Place some extra padding to the middle to make it comfortable for your casualty. The rope can be adjusted to suit the height of the casualty by re-coiling and making the rope shorter or longer.

MOVING AND CARRYING A CASUALTY
WHEN YOU ARE PART OF A GROUP

Basic sheet stretcher

Carrying a stretcher in case of an emergency may not be feasible nor practical, but there are materials which can be used to improvise and construct your own stretcher.

Materials could include:

- Groundsheet / tarpaulin
- Group shelter
- Bivi bag
- Tent
- Survival bag
- Blanket or towels
- Walking poles
- Items of clothing
- Rucksacks
- Branches
- Stones

Lifting technique

1 Let your casualty know what you are about to do. Keep talking to them and provide reassurance

2 A lead First Aider should be appointed to take charge of the lift and are usually positioned at the head

3 Other members of the group should be positioned equally along the sides of the 'stretcher' as close to the casualty as possible

4 Items such as smooth tree branches can be used at each side of the chosen material to act as handles when lifting and carrying. 'Roll' the branches up at each side to act as handles for lifting and carrying

5 The lifting and lowering of your casualty must be synchronised on the lead First Aiders command

6 Make sure all members of the group who are lifting are clear on what they need to do

7 On the command of the lead First Aider, each member of the group lifts at the same time, slowly and smoothly, adopting a good posture with backs straight and knees bent

If you or another member of the group has walking poles and can manage without them, they can act as the handles on each side of the stretcher which are likely to be more stable and trustworthy than items found in the wilderness.

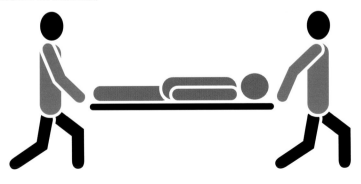

Clothing and walking poles stretcher

If you do not have access to sheet like materials to construct the stretcher, you may be able to use coats or jackets to act as the stretcher base. Zip the jackets up and turn the sleeves inside out. Tape a set of walking poles together length ways so that they are long enough for your casualty – repeat this for the other side of the stretcher.

Feed the taped walking poles through the inverted sleeves. Use the same lifting technique as above for the basic sheet stretcher.

Moving and carrying your casualty on an improvised stretcher will require several people due to the weight of the casualty and the shape of the stretcher. If you suspect a spinal or head injury, pelvic or thigh bone fracture, do not move and carry your casualty using an improvised stretcher - summon for professional medical assistance.

MOVING AND CARRYING A CASUALTY
SUSPECTED SPINAL INJURY

Moving and carrying a casualty who may have sustained a spinal injury needs to be performed with extreme care and attention, as it is possible to make their condition worse. You may need to move the casualty to a safer place to reduce the risk of further injuries and to summon for professional medical help.

1 Ensure the head is fully supported throughout the lifting, carrying and lowering of your casualty

2 Each member of the group crouches down alongside the casualty, grasping hold of their clothing just underneath them to secure the grip ready for lifting

3 Members of the group next to the casualty's legs need to slide their hands underneath both legs

4 On the lead First Aider's command, lift the casualty keeping them as straight and stable as possible, ensuring the head is supported in a neutral position throughout the lift and carry

5 Move very slowly and carefully in the direction of travel and keep the head, neck and spine as straight as possible

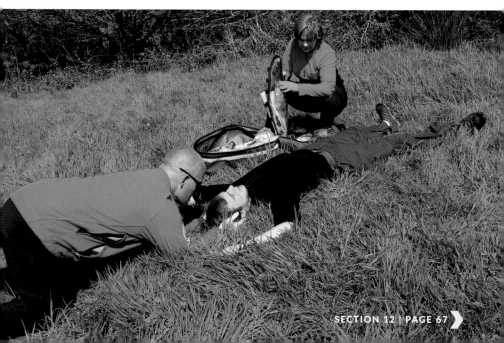

THE SKELETON

The human skeleton is made up of 206 bones, the largest being the femur, or thigh bone. A joint is the connection between bones which are supported in place by ligaments. Muscles around the skeleton create the movement which are connected to the bones via tendons.

The skeleton serves many purposes:

- It protects vital organs such as the brain, heart and lungs
- It supports muscles held to the skeleton by tendons
- It provides movement in the form of joints which are held together by ligaments

There are three types of joints:

1 Non-movable - such as the bones that make up the skull
2 Partially movable - such as the ribs and spine
3 Movable joints - such as the hip, which is made up of a ball and socket

Through various outdoor activities, bones can be damaged or broken.

Breaks or fractures fall into three main categories:

1 Closed fracture. This is where the break does not penetrate the skin
2 Open fracture. This is where the broken bone does penetrate the skin
3 Complicated fracture. This is where the broken bone injures another part of the body i.e. a broken rib penetrating a lung

In respect of first aid, there is nothing you can do to repair a fracture. However, you can offer treatment that will make your casualty more comfortable in order to prevent the injury from worsening.

DO NOT attempt to straighten or realign a fracture.

Your aims are to:

- Prevent movement of the broken bone
- Support them in the position found
- Call the emergency services
- Limit their pain
- Reduce the chance of further injury
- Facilitate safe and prompt transport if practicable

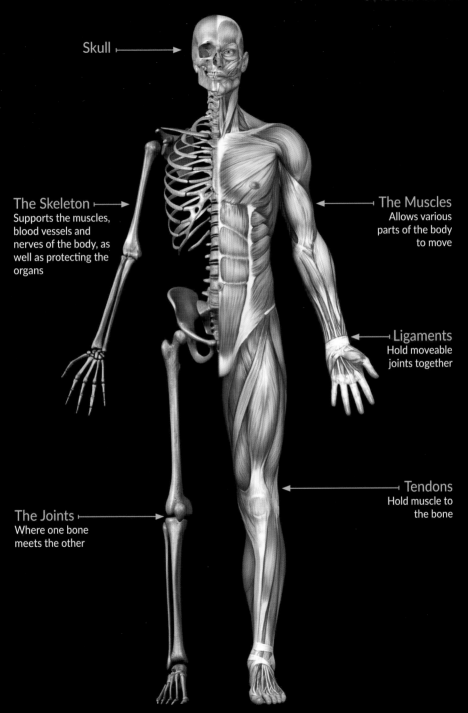

Skull

The Skeleton
Supports the muscles,
blood vessels and
nerves of the body, as
well as protecting the
organs

The Muscles
Allows various
parts of the body
to move

Ligaments
Hold moveable
joints together

Tendons
Hold muscle to
the bone

The Joints
Where one bone
meets the other

CLOSED FRACTURE

Signs and symptoms

- Pain
- Swelling
- Deformity
- Internal bleeding
- Bruising
- Shock

Treatment

- Insulate from the ground and provide shelter if possible
- Immobilise the injured part to stop any movement
- Place padding around the injury for further support
- Leave the casualty in the position found unless they can move the injured part to a more comfortable position
- For additional support, particularly if there is a delay in the emergency services arriving, you could consider strapping an uninjured leg to the injured one. Use broad-fold bandages and ensure that any knots are tied to the uninjured side. Do not wrap a bandage over the fracture. If their circulation is impaired, loosen the dressings
- You MUST NOT try to realign the fracture. This should only be performed by medically trained professionals
- Do not give you casualty anything to eat or drink
- Treat for shock
- Summon for professional help if they are unable to walk

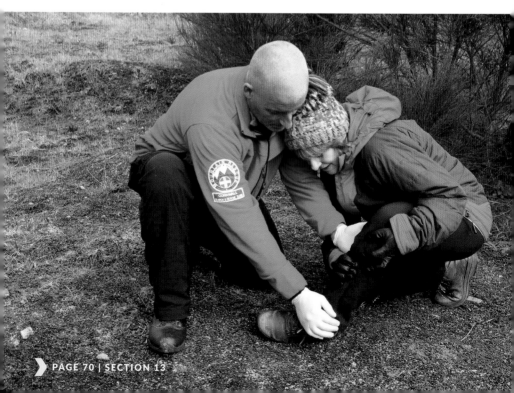

SUPPORT SLING

Fractures to the lower arm and wrist are a common injury. In adults, it accounts for approximately half of all broken bones. In children, fractures of the forearm are second only to broken collarbones.

There is little a First Aider can do other than support it and to dispatch them to hospital for treatment.

In respect of support, generally speaking your casualty will support it themselves, and will not want you to move it. If they are unable to support it themselves, then you can offer to apply a support sling using a triangular bandage.

1. Identify the injury to the arm and providing the arm can be bent at the elbow, offer your casualty a support for it

2. Pass the bandage under the injured arm with the long base running parallel with the body. The point opposite the long base should be at the elbow of the injured arm

3. Bring the lower point of the bandage up over the injured arm and over the shoulder so that the two ends meet

4. Tie off the two ends on the injured side above the collar bone. Place the two ends under the knot to act as a cushion for the knot

5. Secure the trailing bandage at the elbow with a safety pin, or by twisting it fairly tight and losing it by tucking it away within the sling

6. Ensure that there is still circulation in the fingertips by performing a capillary refill check. Press a fingernail which should go pale. When released it should go back to normal colouration

7. Summon for professional medical assistance if they are unable to walk

ELEVATED SLING FOR FOREARM AND HAND INJURIES

1. Ask the casualty to support the injured arm across their chest, with their fingers resting on the opposite shoulder whilst you apply the elevated sling

2. Place the bandage diagonally across the chest from the shoulder, so that the long base is running parallel with the body. One end of the bandage should be placed just over their shoulder on the uninjured side and the point opposite the long base should be at the elbow of the injured arm

3. Tuck the base of the bandage under their hand, forearm and elbow

4. Bring the lower end of the bandage diagonally across their back, to meet the other end at their shoulder. Tie the ends into a knot to secure the bandage.

5. Twist the point of the bandage at the elbow and tuck it in to secure it. If you have a safety pin, this can be used to fasten the point at the corner. Ensure the casualty feels comfortable and bandage is supporting the injured arm

6. Keep their fingers exposed so you can check their circulation at regular intervals. If it is too tight, loosen the bandage and tie again

OPEN FRACTURE

Signs and symptoms

- Pain
- Deformity
- Internal bleeding
- External bleeding
- Shock

Treatment

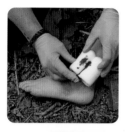

- Call the emergency services
- Prevent any movement
- Reduce the risk of infection by wearing gloves
- Control the blood loss by dressing around the wound
- DO NOT apply any direct pressure on the protruding bone
- Use sterile non-fluffy dressings

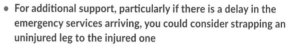

- For additional support, particularly if there is a delay in the emergency services arriving, you could consider strapping an uninjured leg to the injured one
- Use broad-fold bandages and ensure that any knots are tied to the uninjured side
- Do not wrap a bandage over the fracture. If their circulation is impaired, loosen the dressings
- You MUST NOT try to realign the fracture. This should only be performed by medically trained professionals

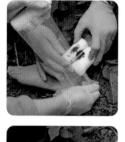

- Treat for shock, insulate from the ground and provide shelter whilst waiting for professional medical help to arrive
- Monitor vital signs at regular intervals
- Do not offer the casualty anything to eat, drink or smoke as a general anaesthetic may have to be administered when they get to hospital

COMPLICATED FRACTURE

Signs and symptoms

- Pain
- Deformity
- Internal and external bleeding
- Shock

Treatment

- Call the emergency services
- Apply the same treatment as mentioned before for an open or closed fracture
- Be aware of a possible secondary injury which may not be visible. An example of this could be a fractured rib which may have affected an internal organ
- Monitor them very closely and be prepared to resuscitate them

IMPROVISED SLINGS AND SPLINTS

The key element of treatment for your casualty with a suspected fracture is to prevent any movement.

It may be difficult to do this in a remote setting due to the lack of equipment, changes to the environment and adverse weather conditions. You may have equipment to hand which can be improvised into a support sling or a splint.

A splint is a piece of equipment used to immobilise an injured body part and protect it from further damage. Splints are often used to stabilise a broken bone before the casualty is taken to hospital to receive more advanced treatment. Splints can also be used for severe sprains and strains.

Materials which you can use to create a sling or splint include:

Sling   Triangular bandage, other first aid bandages, clothing, bicycle inner tube, trouser belt, rucksack straps, tape.

Splint

Splint structure: Walking poles, tent poles, wood, tree branches, plastic sheet, rucksacks, clothing, dressings, padding, tape.

Splint comfort
and support: Bandages, dressings, padding, clothing, towels, rope, string, shoelaces, tape.

Different ways to splint or immobilise a fracture:

- **Fingers**   Thin pad (eye pad dressing) between the finger and taped together
- **Hand**   Immobilise hand and apply arm sling
- **Upper arms**   Arm sling and lots of padding, apply a broad fold bandage carefully to secure
- **Collar Bone**   Immobilise injured side with an elevated sling
- **Elbow**   Arm sling
- **Forearm**   Splint, immobilise, arm sling
- **Wrist**   Splint, immobilise, arm sling
- **Pelvis**   Very carefully pad between and bring the knees together and immobilise
- **Thigh**   Padding between the leg, immobilise to the other leg
- **Lower leg**   Splint independently
- **Ankle**   Splint independently

TENT POLE SPLINT

1 Tape an unassembled tent pole together to form the base of the splint, which provides a good surface area for their arm to rest

2 Place padding on top of the tent poles

3 Ask your casualty to gently rest their arm onto the padding

4 Use a bandage (or similar) to tie around the splint and your casualty's arm to secure it in place

5 Do not overtighten the splint as this could affect the casualty's blood flow and worsen their condition

6 Leave a slight gap at the wrist so that you have access to check their pulse

7 Your casualty's arm should now be splinted securely and comfortably

SAM® SPLINT

(Structural Aluminium Malleable Splint)

The SAM® splint is a commercially available splint that is simple in design, compact and lightweight. It is used for immobilising bone and soft tissue injuries in an emergency setting and will fit perfectly in a good-sized rucksack.

The SAM® splint is quite simply an aluminium sheet completely covered in foam, which serves as padding for the splint. The splint can be adjusted so that it conforms to the limb and then secured with a bandage.

DISLOCATIONS

Dislocations are extremely painful and are often caused by a violent muscle contraction, a strong force wrenching the bone into an abnormal position, or even as something as simple as turning over whilst sleeping can cause it.

The recognition of a dislocation is that of a fracture, with the addition of disfigurement around the joint. In all cases, the ligaments holding the bones together will be damaged. Under no circumstances should you try to put the dislocated joint back into place.

You must send your casualty to hospital for treatment as soon as possible.

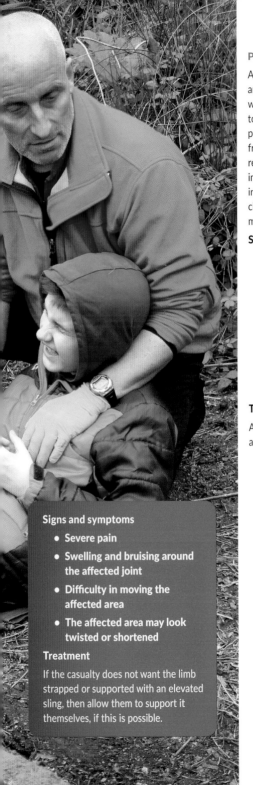

PELVIC INJURIES

Any injury to the pelvis can be life threatening and must be treated with extreme care, especially where the casualty may have sustained a fracture to the pelvis. The femoral arteries run through the pelvis and any form of movement could cause the fractured bone to damage these major blood vessels, resulting in an internal catastrophic bleed. Pelvic injuries are usually associated with major traumatic incidents such as a fall from height whilst rock climbing, a high-speed collision whilst skiing, or a major crush injury from falling cliff debris.

Signs and symptoms

- **Severe pain, swelling and bruising in the groin and hip area**
- **Pain in the lower back, buttocks and abdominal area**
- **Numbness and tingling in the genital area and upper thighs**
- **Bleeding from the rectum, vagina and/or urethra**
- **Inability to stand or walk**

Treatment

Assume the pelvis has been broken and treat as for a fracture.

- **Call the emergency services immediately**
- **DO NOT touch the pelvis. Establish how the injury happened and note the casualty's symptoms to pass on to the emergency services**
- **Control any external bleeding and treat for shock**
- **Immobilise the injury by tying the casualty's legs together at the ankles**
- **Place padding in between their legs and under their knees for support**
- **Insulate the casualty from the ground, provide shelter and keep them warm**
- **Monitor vital signs whilst awaiting professional medical assistance**

Signs and symptoms

- **Severe pain**
- **Swelling and bruising around the affected joint**
- **Difficulty in moving the affected area**
- **The affected area may look twisted or shortened**

Treatment

If the casualty does not want the limb strapped or supported with an elevated sling, then allow them to support it themselves, if this is possible.

SPRAINS AND STRAINS

These are most commonly associated with sports injuries, or when a person moves suddenly and exerts a great deal of pressure on the muscles or joints. It is sometimes difficult to distinguish between the type of soft tissue injury and a fracture because of the pain and swelling. If you are unsure, you should suspect the worse and treat for a fracture.

Sprains and strains are collectively known as soft tissue injuries.

SPRAIN

A sprain occurs when one or more of the ligaments have been stretched, twisted, or torn, usually as a result of excessive force being applied to a joint. The most common locations for a sprain to occur are:

- **The knee - which can become strained when a person turns quickly during sports or other physical activities**
- **The ankle - which can become strained when walking or running on an uneven surface**
- **The wrist - which can become strained when a person falls onto their hand**
- **The thumb - which can become strained during intense and repetitive physical activity, such as playing a racquet sport**

STRAIN

A strain occurs when the muscle fibres stretch or tear.

They usually occur for one of two reasons:

- **When the muscle has been stretched beyond its limits**
- **When the muscle has been forced to contract** (shorten too quickly)

Strains can develop as the result of an accident, or during physical or sporting activities, such as fell walking, cycling or canoeing.

The most common types of strains are:

Hamstring strains - the hamstrings are muscles that run down the back of the leg and are connected to the hip and knee joints

Calf muscle strains - the gastrocnemius and soleus are the medical names for the muscles of the calf located between the ankle and the knee at the back of the leg

Quadriceps strains - the quadriceps are muscles located at the front of the thigh

Lumbar strains - the lumbar muscles are found in the lower back

Signs and symptoms for both sprains and strains

- **Pain**
- **Swelling**
- **Bruising**
- **Inflammation**
- **Cramp** (Strains)

Treatment

Firstly, protect the injury from worsening. Asking the casualty to walk or run off the injury could seriously jeopardise the extent of the injury!

Protect -   the injured area from further injury by using a support or (in the case of an ankle injury) wearing shoes that enclose and support the feet, such as lace-ups. You may need to move the casualty to an appropriate area to administer first aid treatment and to protect them and yourself from any dangers.

Rest -   by stopping the activity that caused the injury and rest the injured joint or muscle. You may need to set-up shelter for the casualty to rest and for protection against the elements. Avoid physical activity for the first 48 to 72 hours after the injury was afflicted.

Ice -   Immediately after the injury, apply an instant ice pack to the affected area for instant pain relief. For the first 48 to 72 hours after the injury, apply ice wrapped in a damp towel to the injured area for 15 to 20 minutes every two to three hours during the day. Do not leave the ice on whilst sleeping, and do not allow the ice to touch the skin directly, because it could cause a cold burn.

Compress -   or bandage the injured area to limit any swelling and movement that could damage it further. Use a simple elastic bandage or elasticated tubular bandage. It should be wrapped snuggly around the affected area, but not so tightly that it restricts blood flow. Remind your casualty to remove the bandage before going to sleep.

Elevation -   keep the injured area raised and supported to help reduce swelling.

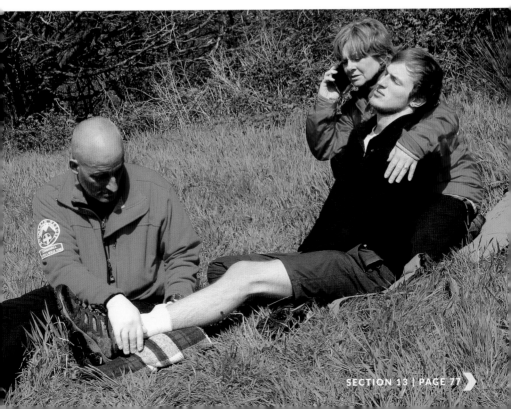

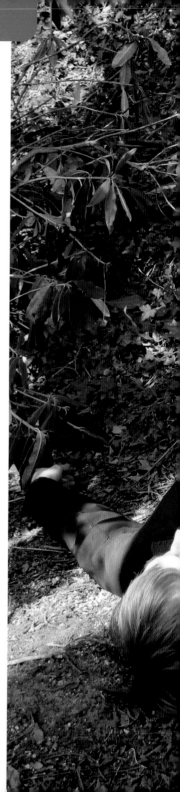

CAUSES OF UNRESPONSIVENESS

If someone is unable to respond to people or activities, then they are deemed as being unresponsive.

Unresponsiveness can be caused by any major illness or injury as well as substance abuse and alcohol. These conditions include head injuries, poisoning, hypothermia, heatstroke, epilepsy, diabetes, heart attack, stroke and shock. This is by no means the definitive list and this section addresses just some of these conditions.

All injuries to the head are potentially dangerous and they all require a medical assessment.

During any assessment of a head injury, or unresponsiveness, it is useful to record and monitor the casualty. You should be monitoring and looking at the following:

- **Eyes**
- **Speech**
- **Movement**
- **Breathing**
- **Responsiveness**

Your objective throughout this monitoring process, is to note any changes in the condition of your casualty in respect of improvement or deterioration. You should continue to monitor your casualty until professional medical help arrives and takes over from you.

CONCUSSION

A concussion is a traumatic brain injury that may result in a bad headache, altered levels of alertness, or unresponsiveness.

It temporarily interferes with the way your brain works, and it can affect memory, judgment, reflexes, speech, balance, coordination and sleep patterns.

Signs and symptoms

The most common signs and symptoms of concussion are:

- **Evidence of a head injury** (blood or bruising)
- **Headache and nausea**
- **Dizziness and loss of balance**
- **Confusion, such as being unaware of your surroundings**
- **Feeling stunned or dazed**
- **Disturbances with vision, such as double vision or seeing "stars" or flashing lights**
- **Difficulties with memory**

Treatment

- If they are responsive, rest them by sitting them down, or lying them down with their head raised and hold a cold compress against the injury. Insulate your casualty from the ground if possible

- Keep them warm and keep talking to them

- Ensure the cold compress stays on the injury for no longer than 20 minutes

- Monitor vital signs

- If they are unresponsive, you must call for an ambulance and support them in the position found

- You must recommend that they seek medical advice, particularly if they develop a headache, feel sick or they sleep more than they would normally do

CERBRAL COMPRESSION

This very serious condition is due to pressure being exerted on the brain from a build-up of blood or fluid, a blood clot, or the brain being depressed as a result of a skull fracture.

This may follow on from concussion either directly, or at some point after their apparent recovery. For this reason, all head injuries must be examined by medical personnel.

Signs and symptoms

- Their response levels will deteriorate, possibly leading to unresponsiveness
- Signs of a recent head injury
- Severe headache
- Weakness and/or paralysis down one side of the face or body
- Flushed face and high temperature

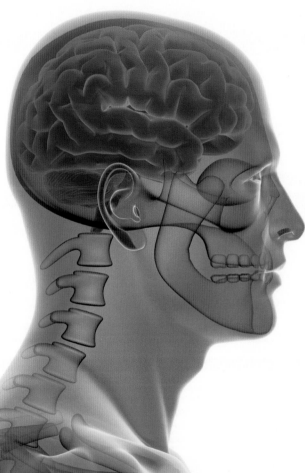

- Drowsiness
- Behavioural changes
- Slow noisy breathing
- Unequal pupil sizes

Treatment

- Call the emergency services immediately by dialling 999/112
- If they are responsive, keep them supported in a comfortable position by lying them down with their head and shoulders raised, providing injuries allow, and keeping them warm
- Monitor their response levels
- If they become unresponsive, check their breathing and carry out your basic life support procedures dependent on the result

SKULL FRACTURE

A skull fracture can be caused by a heavy blow to the head, which may result in a depressed fracture of the skull, or by landing awkwardly from a fall or collision resulting in a base skull fracture. There may also be a wound allowing infection inside the skull. There may also be evidence of concussion and compression.

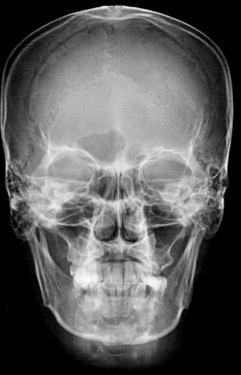

Signs and symptoms

- Evidence of trauma to the head
- Possible depression of the skull
- Bruising around the head
- Clear fluid or watery blood coming from the nose or ear
- Bloodshot eyes
- Deterioration of response levels

Treatment

- If you suspect a spinal injury, do not move them
- Insulate the ground, lay them down, head and shoulders raised if you are able to move them, injured side down
- Call the emergency services immediately
- Monitor vital signs
- Cover their ear with a sterile dressing if there is fluid running out of it
- Control the bleeding and fluid loss
- All head injuries must be advised to go to hospital

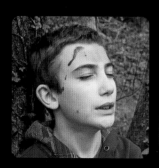
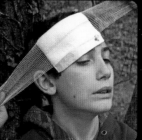
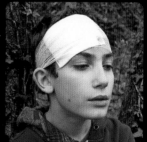

SPINAL INJURIES

The spine, also known as the backbone, is a strong, flexible column of ring-like bones that runs from our skull to our pelvis. It holds the head and body upright and allows us to bend and twist our body. It also offers protection to our spinal cord - a large bundle of nerves that runs through the cavity in the centre of our spine that relays messages between our brain and the rest of our body.

It is made up of 33 irregularly shaped bones called vertebrae. Each vertebra has a hole in the middle through which the spinal cord runs.

The spine can be divided into five different regions, from top to bottom:

1 Seven cervical vertebrae support our head and neck and allow us to nod and shake our head

2 Our ribs are attached to our 12 thoracic vertebrae

3 Our five sturdy lumbar vertebrae carry most of the weight of our upper body and provide a stable centre of gravity when we move

4 Our sacrum is made up of five fused vertebrae. It makes up the back wall of our pelvis

5 Our coccyx is made up of four fused vertebrae. It is an evolutionary remnant of the tail found in most other vertebrates

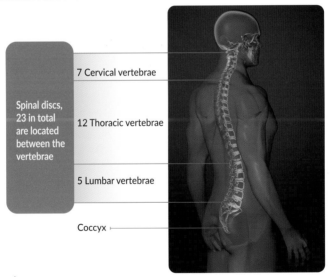

7 Cervical vertebrae

Spinal discs, 23 in total are located between the vertebrae

12 Thoracic vertebrae

5 Lumbar vertebrae

Coccyx

Shock absorbers

Sandwiched between our vertebrae are pads of tough, fibrous cartilage called inter-vertebral discs that cushion our vertebrae and absorb shock. These discs, together with the curved 'S' shape of our spine, prevents shock to our head when we walk or run.

Any damage to our spine can not only be life-threatening, but it can also leave us permanently damaged. It can lead to paralysis to parts of our body that is irreparable.

Therefore, your handling of your casualty where you suspect a spinal injury is critical in ensuring that their condition does not worsen.

Signs and symptoms

When the spinal column or vertebrae are damaged:

- An unusual curvature of the spine
- Pain at the site of injury. Be aware that this may be masked by other pains in other parts of the body
- Tenderness in the skin that covers the spine

When the spinal cord is damaged:

- No control over limb movement
- Loss of sensation, or abnormal sensations such as numbness, burning or tingling
- The casualty may say that the limbs feel heavy or clumsy
- Loss of bladder and bowel control
- Breathing difficulties

Treatment – responsive and breathing normally

- Reassure your casualty and tell them not to move
- Prevent any movement and support in the position found
- Support their head but do not cover their ears with your hands, as this will impair their hearing

    To support their head, kneel or lie down behind their head. Rest your elbows on your knees, or the ground to keep your arms steady. Grip each side of their head without covering their ears and remain in this position so that the head, neck and spine are supported.

- Call the emergency services
- Monitor their breathing and other vital signs whilst you are waiting for professional medical help to arrive
- Take a thorough history of what happened and ask your casualty about their levels of pain, if any. This can be passed on to the emergency services when they arrive
- Be prepared to resuscitate if your casualty stops breathing normally

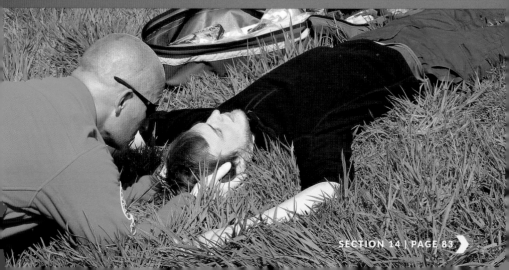

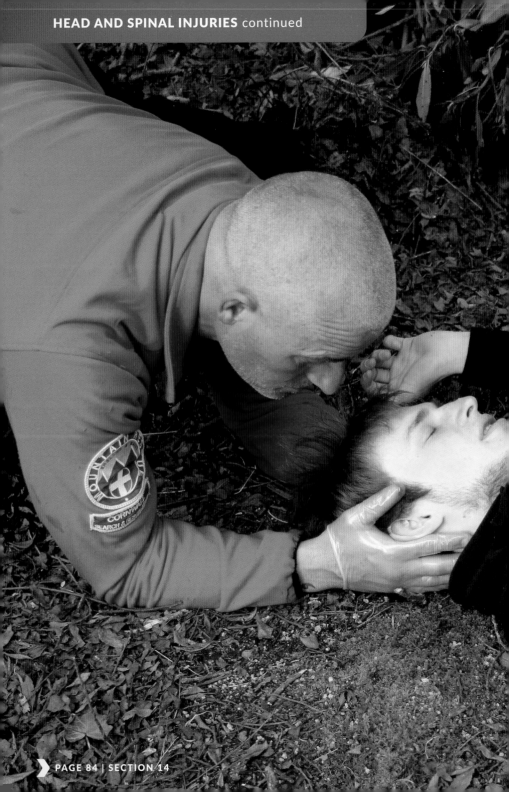

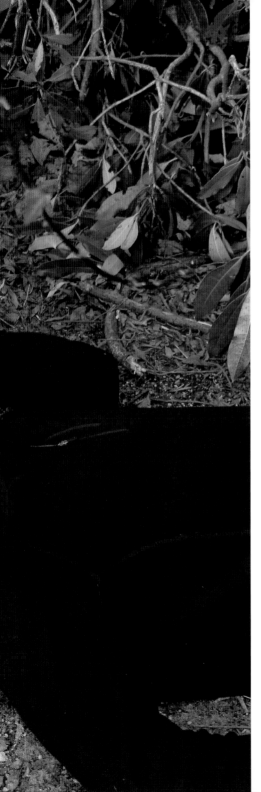

MODIFIED RECOVERY POSITION

If your casualty is unresponsive but breathing normally, it may be necessary to place them into the modified recovery position. This differs from the normal recovery position and ideally, you will require a second person.

- Support the casualty's head and neck by placing your hands either side of their head. The other person should gently raise one leg so it is bent at the knee

- Stretch the casualty's arm out so it is positioned at a right angle from the body. The opposite arm to the leg that is raised should be placed over the casualty's chest area

- The casualty should then be moved gently onto their side. Ensure that they are fully supported and their head is held in line with their spine

- Finally, you should move the top leg and settle the arm under the casualty's cheek. The other person should support the head and neck throughout

If you do not have help to hand, place your casualty into the standard recovery position, whilst trying to keep the spine as straight as possible.

Be prepared to resuscitate if your casualty stops breathing normally.

Contained within the chest cavity is the heart and the lungs. These extremely important organs are protected by a ribcage made up of 12 pairs of ribs and the breastbone (sternum). In addition, the ribcage is of sufficient size to give protection to other vital organs such as the liver and spleen. Any wound to the chest could therefore, cause life-threatening damage. These include, penetrating wounds such as a stabbing or a broken rib. An injury that you may not necessarily see could also inflict major damage to any of these organs, and therefore your prompt and effective treatment is vital in preserving life and in preventing the injury from worsening.

DEFINITION OF A CHEST INJURY

A person with a chest injury has damage to a structure in the chest, caused by an injury. Minor injuries may cause a bruise to the chest, while severe injuries may also damage the lungs or heart.

PENETRATING CHEST WOUNDS

Signs and symptoms

- Obvious signs of trauma – blood loss
- Shortness of breath
- Respiratory distress
- Chest pain
- Shock
- **Cyanosis** (blueness around the extremities such as the ears and lips)
- Swelling
- Chest wall bruising
- Open wounds
- Distended neck veins
- **Tracheal deviation** (shifting of the windpipe)

In addition, you may see evidence of the following:

- 'Bubbling' around the wound
- Coughed up red frothy blood
- The sound of air being sucked in when the casualty breathes

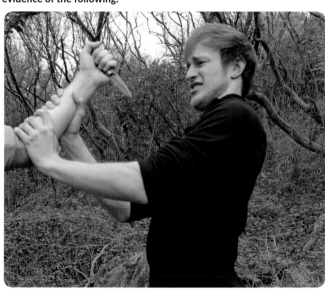

Treatment

- Call the emergency services immediately to request professional medical assistance
- Insulate from the ground, help the casualty to sit down and lean them towards the injured side
- If the wound is bleeding, you must apply direct pressure to the wound and apply a non-occlusive dressing if it is necessary
- If your casualty has a 'sucking' chest wound where you can hear air escaping from the wound, leave the wound exposed to freely communicate with the open environment, or apply a non-occlusive dressing if one is available
- If there is something embedded, build up padding on either side of the object until it is high enough for you to be able to bandage over the top of the object without pressing it further into the wound.
  If you cannot build padding high enough, build around the object with rolled sterile dressings and secure in place to control the loss of blood
- Treat for shock and monitor vital signs until help arrives

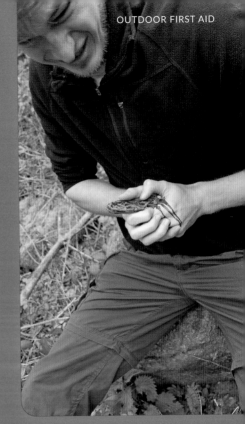

RIBCAGE INJURY

The ribcage can be damaged by a crush, a direct blow to the chest or by falling.

It has been known for a rib to be broken by coughing excessively!

Flail chest is a life-threatening medical condition that occurs when a segment of the rib cage breaks due to trauma and becomes detached from the rest of the chest wall. Two of the symptoms of flail chest are chest pain and shortness of breath.

It is an extremely painful injury, but the concerns are for the vital organs that are contained within the ribcage. Because of this, you may well have to deal with a potentially life-threatening injury such as a punctured lung or internal bleeding.

Treatment

- Sit the casualty down and support them
- Lean them towards the injured side, but comfortably in a position that suits them
- If the casualty allows, apply an elevated sling to the arm on the injured side. Do not enforce this if the injury is so painful that they would prefer to support it themselves
- Call the emergency services
- If the casualty becomes unresponsive, support them in the position found unless you believe their airway is at risk, then you should place them in the recovery position (injured side down), taking extreme care when rolling them over
- Monitor their airway and breathing

CRUSH INJURY

A crush injury occurs when a body part is exposed to a high degree of force, usually after being compressed between two objects. Injuries of this nature can be minor, such as damaging a fingertip while using a mallet to secure your tent, or they can be very serious, such as being crushed by large rocks following an avalanche.

Treatment for casualties that have been crushed for LESS THAN 15 MINUTES

- If it's possible, release the casualty from the crush as soon as you can
- Remember your first aid priorities and treat appropriately
  - Breathing
  - Bleeding
  - Burns and breaks
- Treat for shock and monitor vital signs
- Call the emergency services

Treatment for casualties that have been crushed for MORE THAN 15 MINUTES

- Call the emergency services immediately
- Do not remove the item that is crushing your casualty
- Monitor their breathing and response levels
- Offer them plenty of reassurance
- Treat them for shock

The reason for not releasing the casualty after 15 minutes of being crushed is that toxins will build around the muscle area that is crushed. These potentially life-threatening toxins will be released into the blood stream and that could prove to be fatal.

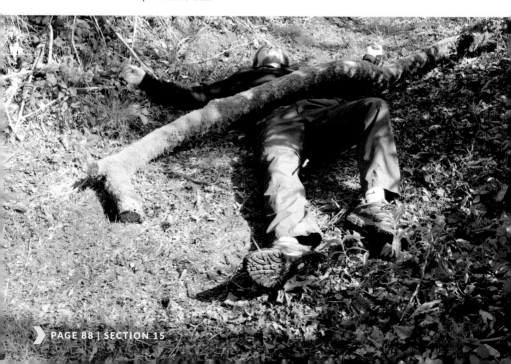

ABDOMINAL INJURIES

Abdominal wounds

If your casualty has been injured by a stabbing, a gunshot or by any other cause that would create a penetrating wound, then your priority is to ensure that your casualty is breathing normally and then to control the blood loss. If there is anything penetrating from the wound such as a knife, then it must be left in place and the wound dressed around it using sterile dressings. It is important to wear gloves as in any type of incident involving blood loss.

Signs and symptoms

- Evidence of blood loss
- Pain
- Possible entry and exit wound with a high velocity wound such as a gunshot
- Shock
- Possible embedded object
- Possible shortness of breath

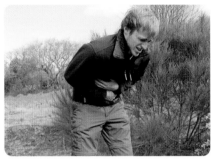

Treatment

- If the casualty is responsive, then lie them down with their knees raised and supported
- Loosen tight clothing
- Dress the wound/s with a sterile dressing and secure it with adhesive tape
- Call the emergency services
- If bloods seeps through the first dressing, then remove it and apply a new one and secure it in place

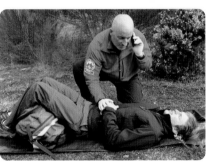

- Treat for shock and monitor their vital signs
- If the casualty becomes unresponsive, support them in the position found unless you believe their airway is at risk, then you should place them in the recovery position (injured side down)

In extreme cases, it is important to ensure that the contents of the abdomen are contained within the abdominal cavity, particularly if the casualty vomits or coughs. Hold a sterile dressing firmly in place over the wound to prevent the contents from spilling out. Be prepared to resuscitate, should they stop breathing normally.

Abdominal pains

Abdominal pains can be brought on by many reasons. In less serious cases, such as stomach ache, then the casualty will normally recover without the intervention of medical assistance. If the pain is severe, and it induces vomiting or diarrhoea, then you should encourage your casualty to visit their GP. If the pain is so severe that it causes the casualty to 'double up' in pain, particularly if the pain comes in 'waves', then you should summon for professional medical assistance.

HEART ATTACK

A heart attack is a serious medical condition in which the supply of blood to the heart is suddenly blocked, usually by a blood clot. The lack of blood to the heart can seriously damage the heart muscles. If left untreated, the muscles will begin to die. The medical term for a heart attack is myocardial infarction.

Most heart attacks occur in people with coronary heart disease (CHD). This is a serious condition in which the arteries become narrowed and hardened by the build-up of clumps of cholesterol, called plaques.

The two arteries that supply the heart are called the coronary arteries. People with hardened and narrowed coronary arteries are said to have coronary heart disease (CHD).

Risk factors for CHD include:

- Smoking
- High-fat diet
- Diabetes
- Being overweight or obesity

Heart attacks are very common and are one of the leading causes of death in England. Each year in England, an estimated 111,000 people have a heart attack. Many heart attacks that lead to death are preventable. This is because most of the risk factors that are listed above can also be prevented.

Most heart attacks occur in people who are over 45 years of age. Men are two to three times more likely to have a heart attack than women.

Signs and symptoms

The symptoms of a heart attack can include:

- Pale blue/grey, cold and clammy skin
- Chest pain. The pain is usually located in the centre of the chest and can feel like a sensation of pressure, tightness or squeezing
- Pain in other parts of the body. It can feel as if the pain is travelling from the chest to the arms (usually the left arm is affected, but it can affect both arms), jaw, neck, back and abdomen
- Shortness of breath and nausea
- An overwhelming sense of anxiety (similar to having a panic attack)
- Feeling light headed
- Vomiting, coughing and wheezing

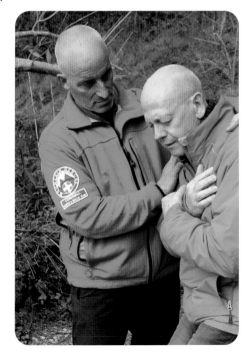

Treatment

- Call the emergency services immediately
- Make your casualty comfortable and insulate them from the ground
- Place the casualty in a reclined sitting position (W) to ease any strain on the heart
- Monitor their vital signs carefully and provide shelter if possible
- Calm and reassure your casualty
- If they become unresponsive, you must open their airway and check for normal breathing, and be prepared to resuscitate them

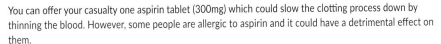

You can offer your casualty one aspirin tablet (300mg) which could slow the clotting process down by thinning the blood. However, some people are allergic to aspirin and it could have a detrimental effect on them.

If you are unsure about the allergy, then DO NOT administer it. You must not administer an aspirin to anyone under the age of 16.

ANGINA

Angina is a heart condition that is caused when the blood supply to the muscles of the heart is restricted. It usually occurs when the arteries that supply the heart become hardened and narrowed.

The main symptom of angina is a dull, heavy or tight pain in the chest that can sometimes spread to the left arm, neck, jaw or back. The pain is usually triggered by physical activity or stress and usually only lasts for a few minutes.

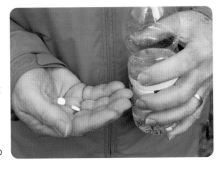

The onset of this type of chest pain is often referred to as an angina attack.

The signs and symptoms are very similar to that of a heart attack, and if you are unsure about their condition, you should offer them treatment as you would for a heart attack victim.

Treating angina

There are three main goals in treating angina. They are:

- To relieve the symptoms during an angina attack by resting and re-assuring them
- To help them administer their own medication such as GTN spray, if they have it
- To call for professional medical assistance if there is no improvement

    Insulate from the ground, set-up shelter and monitor vital signs while awaiting rescue

GTN – glyceryl trinitrate

GTN is used to relieve angina related symptoms. GTN relaxes and widens the blood vessels, which increases oxygen delivery to the heart. GTN can be administered using a spray, tablet or a patch for long term pain control.

STROKE

In simplistic terms, a stroke is a brain attack. A stroke is a serious medical condition that occurs when the blood supply to part of the brain is cut off.

Like all organs, the brain needs the oxygen and nutrients provided by blood to function properly. If the supply of blood is restricted or stopped, brain cells begin to die. This can lead to brain damage and possibly death.

Strokes are a medical emergency and prompt treatment is essential because the sooner your casualty receives treatment for a stroke, the less damage is likely to happen to them.

Types of stroke

There are two main causes of strokes:

- **Ischaemic** (accounting for over 80% of all cases): the blood supply is stopped due to a blood clot
- **Haemorrhagic:** a weakened blood vessel supplying the brain bursts and causes brain damage

There is also a related condition known as a transient ischaemic attack (TIA), where the supply of blood to the brain is temporarily interrupted, causing a 'mini-stroke'. TIA's should be treated as being serious as they are often a warning sign that a stroke is coming.

Strokes can damage:

- **Bodily functions**
- **Our ability to learn**
- **Our thought processes**
- **How we feel and communicate**

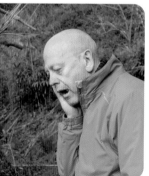

If you suspect a stroke – act **FAST** and call 999/112 for the emergency services. **Stroke is a medical emergency.**

By calling for medical help early, treatment can be given which can prevent further brain damage.

F **Facial weakness**
Can the person smile? Has their mouth or eye drooped?

A **Arm weakness**
Can the person raise both arms?

S **Speech problems**
Can the person speak clearly and understand what you say?

T **Time** to call the emergency services

Treatment

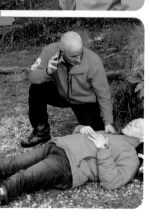

- **Call the emergency services**
- **If the casualty is responsive, lay them down and raise their head and shoulders. Insulate them from the ground and provide shelter**
- **Turn their head to one side, affected side down**
- **If the casualty is unresponsive, place them in the recovery position injured side down**
- **Loosen tight clothing and make your casualty comfortable**
- **Reassure your casualty and monitor vital signs. Be prepared to resuscitate if they stop breathing normally**

DIABETES

Diabetes is a long-term condition caused by too much glucose, a type of sugar, in the blood. It is also known as diabetes mellitus.

Normally, the amount of sugar in the blood is controlled by a hormone called insulin. Insulin is produced by the pancreas, a gland located behind the stomach. When food is digested and enters the bloodstream, insulin helps move any glucose out of the blood and into cells, where it is broken down to produce energy.

For people with diabetes, the body is unable to break down glucose into energy. This is because there is either not enough insulin to move the glucose, or because the insulin that is there does not work properly.

There are two types of diabetes:
type 1 and type 2 diabetes.

Type 1 diabetes occurs when the body produces no insulin. It is often referred to as insulin-dependent diabetes. It is also sometimes known as juvenile diabetes or early-onset diabetes because it usually develops before the age of 40, often during the teenage years.

Type 2 diabetes occurs when not enough insulin is produced by the body for it to function properly, or when the body's cells do not react to insulin. This is called insulin resistance. It is far more common than type 1. Around 90% of all adults in the UK with diabetes have type 2.

General signs and symptoms

- Feeling very thirsty
- Going to the toilet a lot, especially at night
- Extreme tiredness
- Weight loss and muscle wasting (loss of muscle bulk)

Hyperglycaemia occurs when there is a higher than normal level of glucose (sugar) in the blood.

This causes:

- Increased thirst
- The need to urinate frequently
- Tiredness

Hypoglycaemia means that there is an abnormally low level of sugar (glucose) in the blood.

When the glucose level is too low – called a 'hypo' – the body does not have enough energy to carry out its activities.

Most people will have some warning that their blood glucose levels are too low, which will give them time to correct it.

Typical early warning signs are:

- Feeling hungry
- Trembling or shakiness
- Sweating

DIABETES continued ...

Treatment

Hyperglycaemia

- Call the emergency services immediately
- Insulate your casualty from the ground, provide shelter and monitor vital signs carefully
- If they become unresponsive, place them in the recovery position

Treatment

Hypoglycaemia

- Insulate your casualty from the ground and sit them down
- Offer them 15-20gms of glucose. Offer a sugary drink or sweet food if glucose is not available
- Monitor, comfort and reassure your casualty
- Call the emergency services if the above is ineffective
- If they become unresponsive, place them in the recovery position and continue to monitor vital signs

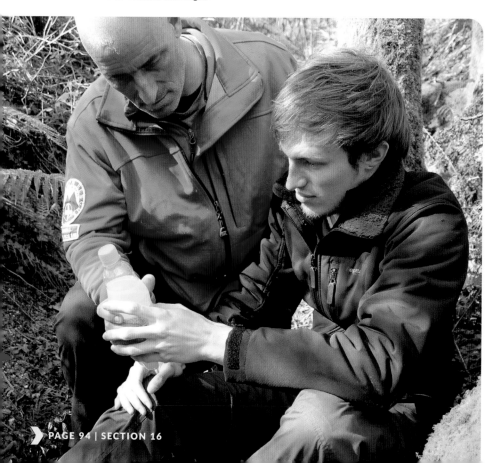

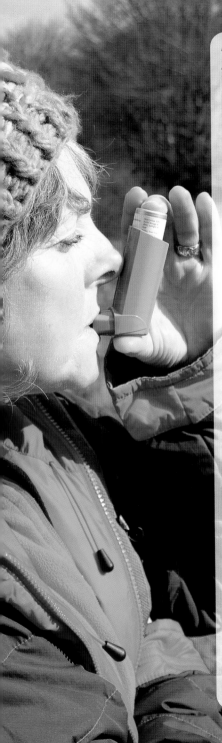

ASTHMA

Asthma is caused by an inflammation to the airways, and in particular the small tubes, called bronchi, which carry air in and out of the lungs. For those who have asthma, the bronchi will be inflamed and more sensitive than normal.

When they come into contact with something that irritates their lungs, known as a trigger, their airways become narrow, the muscles around them tighten and there is an increase in the production of sticky mucus (phlegm).

This makes it difficult to breathe and causes wheezing and coughing. It may also make their chest feel tight.

A severe onset of symptoms is known as an asthma attack. Asthma attacks may require hospital treatment and can sometimes be life-threatening, although this is rare.

For some people with chronic (long-lasting) asthma, long-term inflammation of the airways may lead to more permanent narrowing.

Signs and symptoms

- **Difficulty in breathing**
- **Wheezing**
- **Distress and anxiety**
- **Difficulty in speaking**
- **Grey/blue skin tones**
- **May become exhausted**
- **Coughing**

Treatment

- **Alleviate their concerns by calming them and offering plenty of support and reassurance**
- **Make them comfortable and relaxed by sitting them down**
- **Allow them to use their own inhaler**
- **Insulate from the ground, provide shelter and monitor vital signs, particularly their breathing**
- **Be prepared to resuscitate if your casualty stops breathing**

Summon for professional medical help if:

- **The medication has no effect after 5 minutes**
- **If it's the first attack**
- **Breathlessness makes talking difficult**

SEIZURES

What is epilepsy?

Epilepsy is a condition that affects the brain. When someone has epilepsy, it means they have a tendency to have epileptic seizures.

Anyone can have a one-off seizure, but this doesn't always mean they have epilepsy. Epilepsy is usually only diagnosed if someone has had more than one seizure, and doctors think it is likely they could have more.

Epilepsy can start at any age and there are many different types. Some types of epilepsy last for a limited time and the person eventually stops having seizures. But for many people epilepsy is a life-long condition.

What are epileptic seizures?

A seizure happens when there is a sudden burst of intense electrical activity in the brain. This causes a temporary disruption to the way the brain normally works.

The result is an epileptic seizure.

There are many different types of seizure. What happens to someone during a seizure depends on which part of their brain is affected. During some types of seizure, the person may remain alert and aware of what's going on around them, and with other types they may lose awareness. They may have unusual sensations, feelings, or movements, or they may go stiff, fall to the floor and jerk.

WHAT CAUSES EPILEPSY?

Possible causes of epilepsy include:

- **Stroke**
- **A brain infection, such as meningitis**
- **Severe head injury**
- **Problems during birth which caused the baby to get less oxygen**

But in over half of all people with epilepsy, doctors don't know what caused it. Some may have a family history of epilepsy, suggesting that they may have inherited it.

Tonic-clonic seizures are the type of seizure most people recognise.

Someone having a tonic-clonic seizure goes stiff, loses responsiveness, falls to the floor and begins to jerk or convulse. They may go blue around the mouth due to irregular breathing. Sometimes they may lose control of their bladder or bowels, and bite their tongue or the inside of their mouth.

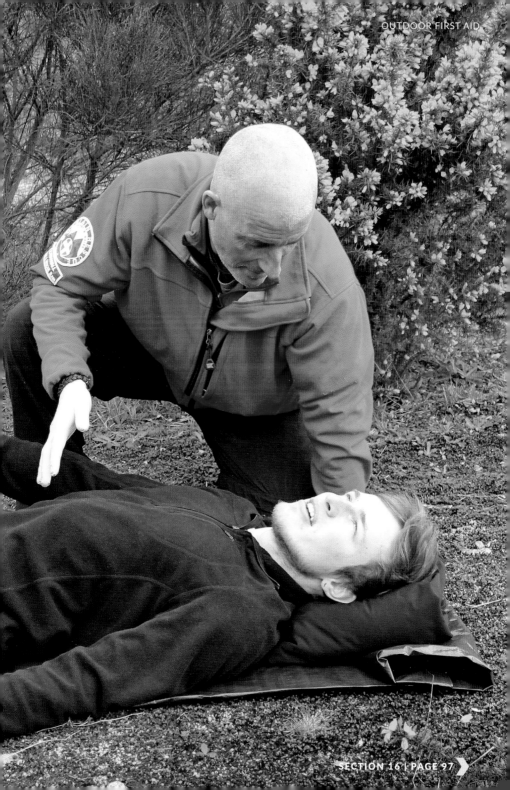

HOW TO HELP IF YOU SEE SOMEONE HAVING A TONIC-CLONIC SEIZURE

Do:

- **Protect them from injury** (remove harmful objects from nearby)
- **Cushion their head**
- **Look for an epilepsy identity card or identity jewellery – it may give you information about their seizures and what to do**
- **Time how long the jerking lasts**
- **Aid breathing by gently placing them in the recovery position once the jerking has stopped**
- **Stay with the them until they are fully recovered**
- **Be calmly reassuring**

Don't:

- **Restrain their movements**
- **Put anything in their mouth**
- **Try to move them unless they are in danger**
- **Give them anything to eat or drink until they are fully recovered**
- **Attempt to bring them round**

Call the emergency services if:

- **You know it is their first seizure**

  or
- **The jerking continues for more than five minutes**

  or
- **They have one tonic-clonic seizure after another without regaining responsiveness between seizures**

  or
- **They are injured during the seizure**

  or
- **You believe they need urgent medical attention**

FOCAL SEIZURES

This type of seizure can also be called a partial seizure. Someone having a focal seizure may not be aware of their surroundings or what they are doing. They may have unusual movements and behaviour such as plucking at their clothes, smacking their lips, swallowing repeatedly or wandering around.

How to help if you see someone having a focal seizure.

Do:

- **Guide them away from danger** (such as open water)
- **Stay with them until recovery is complete**
- **Be calmly reassuring**
- **Explain anything that they may have missed**

Don't:

- **Restrain them**
- **Act in a way that could frighten them, such as making abrupt movements or shouting at them**
- **Assume they are aware of what is happening, or what has happened**
- **Give them anything to eat or drink until they are fully recovered**
- **Attempt to bring them round**

Call the emergency services if:

- **You know it is their first seizure**

  or
- **The seizure continues for more than five minutes**

  or
- **They are injured during the seizure or**
- **You believe they need urgent medical attention**

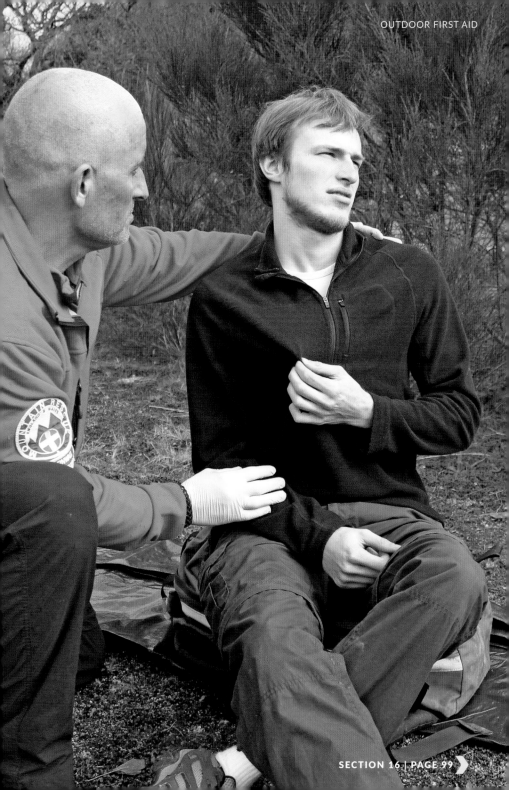

Any allergic reaction including the most extreme form, anaphylactic shock, occurs because the body's immune system reacts inappropriately in response to the presence of a substance that it wrongly perceives as a threat.

An anaphylactic reaction is caused by the sudden release of chemical substances, including histamine, from cells in the blood and tissues where they are stored. The release is triggered by the reaction between the allergic antibody (IgE) and the substance (allergen) causing the anaphylactic reaction. This mechanism is so sensitive that minute quantities of the allergen can cause a reaction. The released chemicals react on blood vessels to cause the swelling in the mouth and anywhere on the skin. There is a fall in blood pressure and, in asthmatics; the effect is mainly on the lungs.

What can cause anaphylaxis?

Common causes include foods such as peanuts, tree nuts (e.g. almonds, walnuts, cashews, Brazils), sesame, fish, shellfish, dairy products and eggs. Non-food causes include wasp or bee stings, natural latex (rubber), penicillin or any other drug or injection. For some people, exercise can trigger a severe reaction - either on its own or in combination with other factors such as food or drugs (e.g. aspirin). Likely causes of anaphylaxis in the outdoor environment apart from food stuffs will include wasp and bee stings, as well as snake bites.

Signs and symptoms

The symptoms of anaphylaxis usually start between 3 and 60 minutes after contact with the allergen. Less commonly, they can occur a few hours or even days after contact.

When your casualty has an anaphylactic reaction, they may feel unwell or dizzy or may faint because of a sudden drop in blood pressure.

Narrowing of the airways can also occur at the same time, with or without the drop in blood pressure. This can cause breathing difficulties and wheezing.

Your casualty may also experience any of the symptoms below:

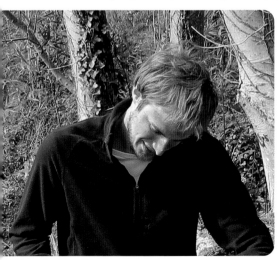

- Swollen eyes, lips, hands, feet and other areas
- A strange metallic taste in the mouth
- Sore, red, itchy eyes
- Changes in heart rate
- A sudden feeling of extreme anxiety or apprehension
- Itchy skin or nettle-rash (hives)
- Unresponsiveness due to very low blood pressure
- Abdominal cramps, vomiting or diarrhoea
- Nausea and fever

Your casualty would not necessarily experience all of these symptoms.

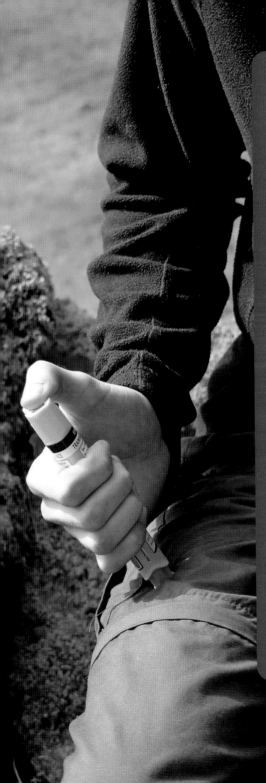

Adrenaline is the gold standard in the treatment of anaphylaxis, and its administration should not be delayed.

In a first aid situation, adrenaline will normally be delivered by an auto-injector.

If available, an injection of adrenaline should be given as soon as possible.

If after 5 minutes the casualty still feels unwell, a second injection should be given.
This should be given in the opposite thigh.

A second dose may also be required if the symptoms reoccur.

When treating a potential anaphylactic casualty, it should be noted that there are NO contraindications for the use of adrenaline.

Treatment for a severe reaction

- **Use an adrenaline auto-injector if the person has one**
- **Call the emergency services (even if they start to feel better) – mention that you think the person has anaphylaxis**
- **Lie the person down flat – unless they are unresponsive, pregnant or having breathing difficulties**
- **Give another injection after 5 minutes if the symptoms do not improve and a second auto-injector is available. This should be given in the opposite thigh**
- **If they become unresponsive, check that their airway is open and clear, and they are breathing normally**
- **Place them in the recovery position**
- **Insulate from the ground, provide shelter and monitor vital signs**
- **Be prepared to resuscitate if they stop breathing normally**

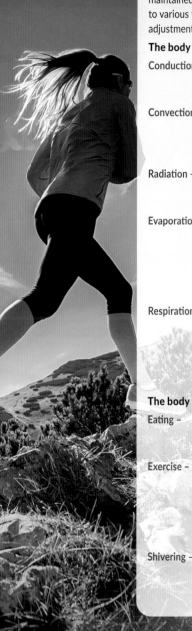

BODY TEMPERATURE CONTROL

The body's 'thermostat' (hypothalamus) is the processing centre in the brain that controls our body temperature. It enables the body temperature to be maintained at a level of around 37 degrees celsius. The hypothalamus responds to various temperature receptors located throughout the body and makes adjustments to maintain a constant core temperature.

The body loses heat by:

Conduction – Losing heat through physical contact with another object or body. For example; sleeping on cold ground, the heat will be transferred from the body to the ground surface.

Convection – Losing heat through the movement of air or water across the skin. For example; the movement of air blowing onto exposed body parts. If the wind is particularly cold, body heat will be lost rapidly through the convection process.

Radiation – Radiation is a form of heat loss through infrared rays. The heat is lost from the body to its surroundings in order to control the body's core temperature.

Evaporation – The process of losing heat through the conversion of water to gas (evaporation of sweat). When we move around and exercise our body, our core body temperature rises and we begin to sweat in an attempt to cool down. The sweat on our skin is evaporated into the air which in turn, cools the surface of our skin.

Respiration – When we breathe, cold air is inhaled from the atmosphere into our lungs. As oxygen is transferred in to the bloodstream and carbon dioxide is transferred out, our body warms the air. When we exhale, warm air is then released into the surrounding environment. Heat loss through respiration is a combination of convection and evaporation.

The body produces heat by:

Eating – When we consume food, our body temperature will increase due to a variety of chemical reactions taking place in our digestive system.

Exercise – During exercise, a series of chemical reactions take place within our muscles which causes them to warm up. The heat produced from exercising our muscles causes our blood vessels to dilate, increasing the blood flow to the skin. Excess heat is lost at the surface area of the skin and released into the surrounding air.

Shivering – Receptors in our skin can detect a drop in core body temperature. Once detected, it triggers our body to shiver. This shivering motion produces heat in an attempt to restore our core body temperature.

HYPOTHERMIA

Hypothermia occurs when a person's normal body temperature of around 37°C (98.6°F) drops below 35°C (95°F).

It is usually caused by being in a cold environment. It can be triggered by a combination of things, including prolonged exposure to cold (such as staying outdoors in cold conditions for a long period of time), rain, wind, sweat, inactivity or being in cold water.

SIGNS AND SYMPTOMS

The symptoms of hypothermia depend on how cold the environment is and how long your casualty is exposed for.

Severe hypothermia needs urgent medical treatment in hospital. Shivering is a good guide to how severe the condition is. If the person can stop shivering on their own, the hypothermia is mild, but if they cannot stop shivering, it is moderate to severe.

Mild cases	Moderate cases	Severe cases
Shivering	Violent, uncontrollable shivering	Loss of control of hands, feet, and limbs
Feeling cold	Being unable to think or pay attention	Uncontrollable shivering that suddenly stops
Low energy	Confusion (some people don't realise they are affected)	Unresponsiveness
Cold, pale skin	Loss of judgement and reasoning	Shallow or no breathing
	Difficulty moving around or stumbling (weakness)	Weak, irregular or no pulse
	Feeling afraid	Stiff muscles
	Memory loss	Dilated pupils
	Fumbling hands and loss of coordination	
	Drowsiness	
	Slurred speech	
	Slow, shallow breathing and a weak pulse	

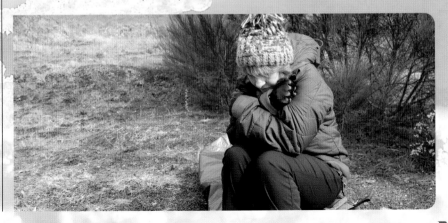

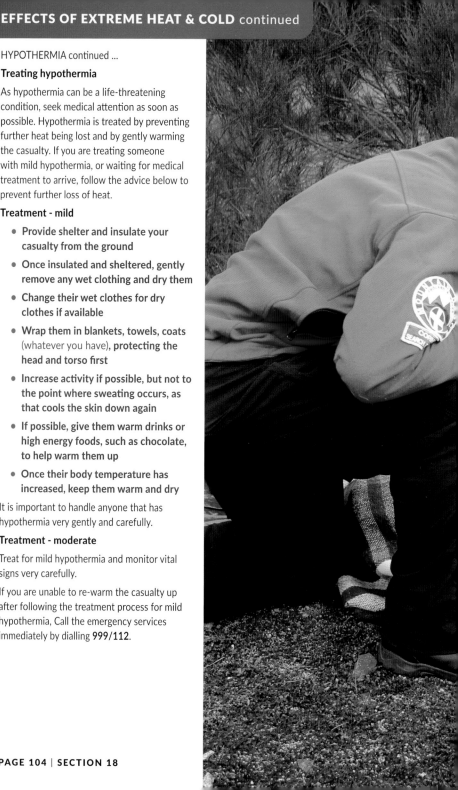

HYPOTHERMIA continued ...

Treating hypothermia

As hypothermia can be a life-threatening condition, seek medical attention as soon as possible. Hypothermia is treated by preventing further heat being lost and by gently warming the casualty. If you are treating someone with mild hypothermia, or waiting for medical treatment to arrive, follow the advice below to prevent further loss of heat.

Treatment - mild

- Provide shelter and insulate your casualty from the ground
- Once insulated and sheltered, gently remove any wet clothing and dry them
- Change their wet clothes for dry clothes if available
- Wrap them in blankets, towels, coats (whatever you have), **protecting the head and torso first**
- Increase activity if possible, but not to the point where sweating occurs, as that cools the skin down again
- If possible, give them warm drinks or high energy foods, such as chocolate, to help warm them up
- Once their body temperature has increased, keep them warm and dry

It is important to handle anyone that has hypothermia very gently and carefully.

Treatment - moderate

Treat for mild hypothermia and monitor vital signs very carefully.

If you are unable to re-warm the casualty up after following the treatment process for mild hypothermia, Call the emergency services immediately by dialling **999/112.**

Treatment – severe

Cases of severe hypothermia require urgent medical treatment in hospital. You should call for professional medical assistance if you suspect your casualty has a case of severe hypothermia.

- **Handle your casualty very gently and carefully**
- **Provide shelter and insulate your casualty from the ground**
- **Place them into the recovery position and monitor vital signs**

Do not give them any food or drink. As the body temperature drops, shivering will stop completely. The heart rate will slow and your casualty will gradually lose responsiveness. Be prepared to resuscitate if they stop breathing normally.

THINGS YOU SHOULD NOT DO

- **Do not apply direct heat** (hot water or a heating pad, for example) **to the arms and legs, as this forces cold blood back to the major organs, making the condition worse**
- **Do not give them alcohol to drink, as this will decrease the body's ability to retain heat**
- **Do not rub or massage their skin, as this can cause the blood vessels to widen and decrease the body's ability to retain heat. In severe cases of hypothermia there is also a risk of heart attack**

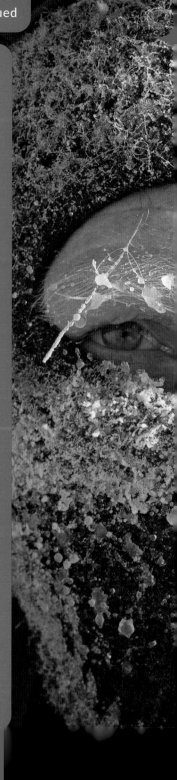

FROSTBITE

Frostbite is a type of cold injury in which the skin and body tissue becomes damaged due to exposure to freezing temperatures.

Frostbite can affect any part of the body, but mainly the extremities such as the hands, feet, ears, nose and lips are affected because they are further away from the body's core, and therefore, have less blood flow.

Early stage - frostnip

Frost nip is the term used for the early stages of frostbite, where your casualty experiences throbbing and aching in the affected area and their skin will become cold, numb and white.

Frostnip treatment

Basic re-warming of the affected area using one's own body heat.

- **Tuck hands under armpits/groin to re-warm**
- **Cover ears, nose or face with dry hands or an item of clothing to re-warm**
- **Breathe onto the affected area through cupped hands to re-warm**

Re-warming the frost nipped area can be very painful for your casualty. Reassure and comfort them until the treatment has been successful and pain levels start to ease.

Never massage the affected area has this can cause further damage.

Intermediate stage – mild frostbite

After the early stages of frostbite, prolonged exposure to cold temperatures will cause more tissue damage and the affected area will feel hard and frozen. Once the tissues have thawed, the skin will turn red and blister.

Mild frostbite treatment

- **Insulate from the ground and provide shelter from the elements**
- **Treat your casualty for hypothermia**
- **Re-warm the affected area slowly using the body's own heat for at least 30 minutes** (see frostnip treatment above)
  If you have warm water available, immerse the affected body part in warm water for at least 30-minutes, until the affected area becomes red-purple in colour and can easily be moved

Advanced stage - deep frostbite

If the affected area continues to be exposed to the cold, the skin may become white, blue or blotchy, and the tissue underneath feels hard and cold to touch. Further damage can occur beneath the skin and affect muscles, tendons, nerves and bones. This stage is also known as 'deep frostbite' and will require urgent medical treatment.

When the skin starts to thaw, blisters will form and turn into thick black scabs. At this stage, it is likely that some tissue will die and will need to be removed to prevent infection.

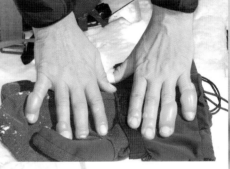

Deep frostbite treatment

- Insulate from the ground and provide shelter from the elements
- Do not attempt any further re-warming
- Remove any jewellery from the affected area
- Dry the affected area and apply a non-absorbent dressing
- Do not try and thaw the injury as it may cause further damage at this stage of frostbite
- Treat for hypothermia
- Summon for professional medical help if you are unable to self-evacuate without causing further tissue damage

HYPERTHERMIA

Hyperthermia is the collective term used to describe several conditions that can occur when the body's core temperature rises above normal. The rise in body temperature is due to the heat-regulating mechanisms failing in our body.

Precautions:

- Reduce levels of exercise during the hottest part of the day
- Be mindful of the temperature
- Stay hydrated and drink plenty of water at regular intervals
- Wear a sunhat and loose clothing
- Remove excess clothing if necessary
- Keep shaded whilst resting
- Avoid alcohol consumption

HEAT EXHAUSTION

Heat exhaustion is brought on when the body's core temperature rises from the normal 37°C up to 40°C (98.6-104°F). At that temperature, the levels of water and salt in the body begin to drop. This causes symptoms such as nausea, feeling faint and heavy sweating.

If it is left untreated, heat exhaustion can sometimes lead to heatstroke. (see opposite page)

Signs and symptoms

- Pale, clammy skin
- Heavy sweating
- Dizziness
- Fatigue
- Nausea
- Vomiting
- Rapid heartbeat
- Mental confusion
- Urinating less often and the colour of the urine being much darker than usual

Treatment

- Get them to rest in the shade with a cool breeze
- Give them plenty of fluids to drink. This should either be water or a rehydration drink such as a sports drink. Avoid alcohol or caffeine as this can increase dehydration
- Cool their skin directly with cold water, or apply wet towels to their skin
- Loosen any unnecessary clothing

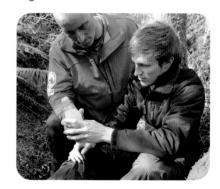

HEATSTROKE

Heatstroke happens when a person's core temperature rises above 40°C (104°F). Cells inside the body begin to break down and important parts of the body stop working.

Symptoms of heatstroke can include mental confusion, hyperventilation (rapid shallow breathing) and loss of responsiveness.

Heatstroke is a medical emergency. If left untreated, it can cause multiple organ failure, brain damage and death.

Signs and symptoms

- **High body temperature: having a temperature of 40°C (104°F) or above is a major sign of heatstroke**
- **Hot and dry skin**
- **Not sweating even while feeling too hot**
- **Rapid heartbeat**
- **Rapid breathing**
- **Muscle cramps**

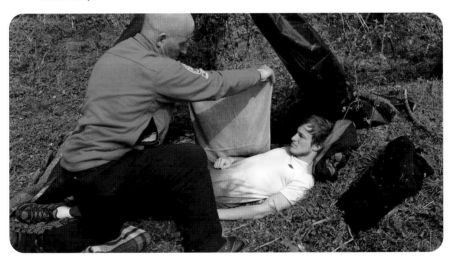

Treatment

- **Move your casualty to a cool area as quickly as possible**
- **If they are responsive, give them water to drink but do not give them any medication**
- **Cover their body with cool, damp towels or sheets, or immerse in cool water**
- **Gently massage their skin to encourage circulation**
- **If seizures start, move nearby objects out of the way to prevent injury** (do not use force or put anything in their mouth)
- **If your casualty is unresponsive and vomiting, place them in the recovery position**
- **Call the emergency services**
- **Monitor vital signs until professional help arrives**

DEHYDRATION

Dehydration is when your body loses more fluids than it can take in. During exercise, fluid is lost predominantly through sweating, so you will need to ensure you drink plenty of fluids before, during and after exercising.

Do not be misled into thinking dehydration only occurs when you are in a hot environment – it is also possible to become dehydrated in cooler temperatures.

Signs and symptoms

- Increased thirst
- Dry mouth and lips
- Dizziness and confusion
- Having dark coloured, strong smelling urine
- Passing urine less often than usual

Treatment

- Stop physical activity
- Rest in the shade with a cool breeze
- Drink plenty of fluids
- Avoid alcohol and caffeine
- Loosen or remove any unnecessary clothing
- Continue to rehydrate throughout the day

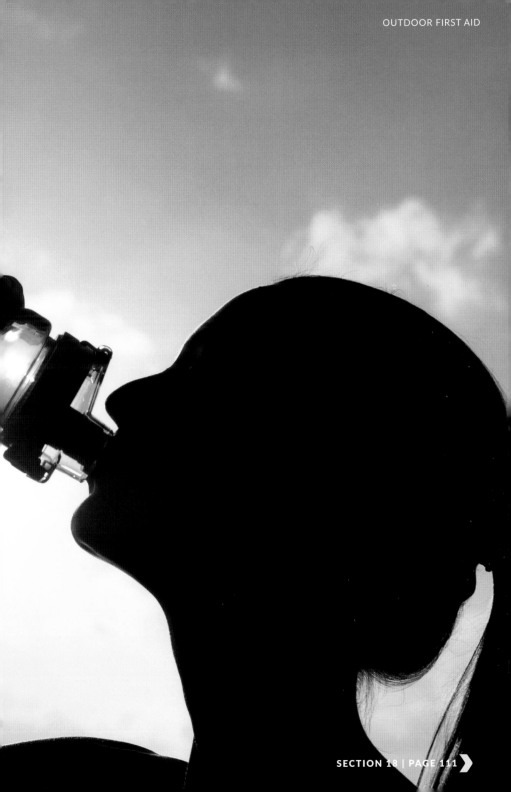

CLASSIFICATION OF BURNS

Burns and scalds are among the most serious and painful of injuries. Burn injuries in the outdoor environment could be caused by naked flames from a camp fire, steam from a boiling kettle, radiation from the sun in the form of ultraviolet (UV) rays and even chemicals used in agricultural work can cause significant burn injuries.

Superficial

The outer layer of skin is burnt causing redness, tenderness and inflammation. Typical factors causing this would be sunburn or touching a hot stove. The skin is not broken or blistered.

Partial thickness

The outer layer of the skin is burnt and broken causing blistering, swelling, pain and rawness.

Full thickness

All the layers of skin have been damaged causing the skin to look pale, charred and waxy with fatty deposits. There may also be damage to the nerves.

When to send a casualty to hospital

Every year in the UK, around 175,000 people attend hospital accident and emergency departments for burn injuries. People who may be at greater risk from the effects of burns, such as children under five years of age and pregnant women, should seek medical attention after a burn or scald.

Assessing the extent of the burn

One quick way to estimate the surface area that has been burned is to compare it to the size of the palm of the casualty's hand, which is roughly equal to 1% of the body's total surface area.

For other groups, you must send them to hospital if:

- The burns affect the hands, feet, face and genital areas
- Full thickness burns
- Burns that extend around a limb
- All partial thickness burns larger than 1% of the body's surface. The casualty's hand represents about 1% on the body's surface
- All superficial burns that represent 5% of the body's surface
- Burns with a mixed pattern of depth

If you are in any doubt, then you should seek medical advice.

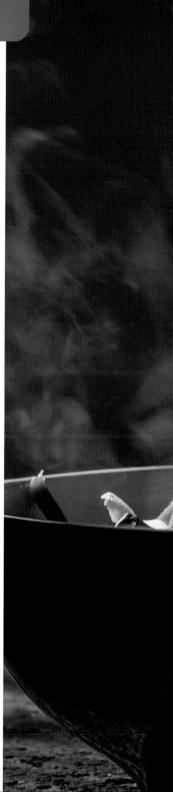

TYPES OF BURNS

Contact burn

As the name suggests, this type of burn occurs when the skin makes contact with a hot object or surface, such as a hot kettle or wood from a burning fire.

Flame burn

This type of burn occurs when naked flames make contact directly with the skin, or where clothing is ignited resulting in the flames and burning material melting on to the skin.

Scald

A scald is caused by hot liquids being spilt onto the skin, such as boiling water from a kettle. The resulting burn injury is usually much worse when it has been caused by steam, as it is hotter than the boiling water itself.

Sun burn

Sunburn is a form of radiation burn that damages the skin through ultraviolet (UV) rays. The skin becomes red in colour, sore and tender to touch, but it can also be more severe, resulting in the skin blistering and swelling, and can contribute towards heatstroke.

You can reduce the risk of being sunburnt by covering up with suitable clothing and applying sunscreen regularly. You can also burn in cool and cloudy conditions, and also from sunlight reflecting off snow.

Ice burn

This is where something that is very cold comes into contact with the skin. Prolonged exposure to cold weather conditions can cause ice burns, and even very cold, high velocity wind can cause the skin to burn.

Friction burn

A friction burn is a form of abrasion caused by the friction of the skin rubbing against a hard surface. Friction burns can occur in activities such as rock climbing, where the rope is run quickly through the hands causing heat to build.

Chemical burn

Chemical burns can occur when an acid or alkali makes contact with the skin or eyes. Chemicals can cause adverse reactions on the body and can even damage internal organs if ingested.

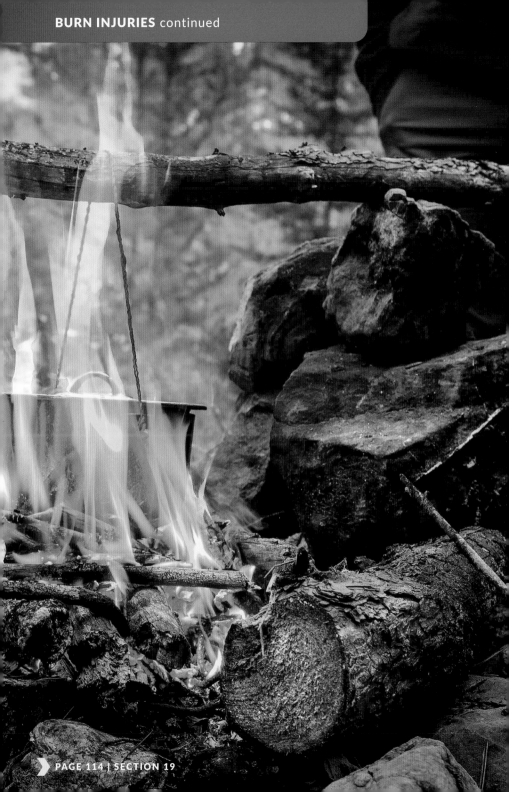

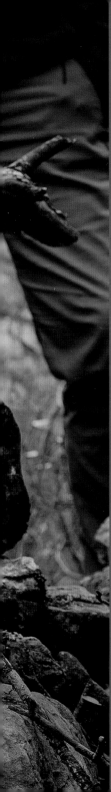

TREATMENT OF BURNS

General treatment of burns

- Ensure the area is safe, particularly from the source that created the burn or scald
- Wear disposable gloves
- Remove clothing, watches and jewellery if it is covering or close to the affected area. Only remove clothing if you are confident it has not stuck to the skin, as this can cause further damage
- Cool the burn with cool running water for 20 minutes using a source of clean water, such as bottled drinking water, or clean running water from a watercourse
- Cover the burn with a suitable sterile dressing or with cling film if you have no appropriate dressing. Burns dressings can also be used which are impregnated with a soothing gel to help relieve pain and to minimise the risk of further tissue damage
- Treat your casualty for shock and monitor vital signs

If the burn injury is very serious:

- Dial 999/112 to request professional medical assistance
- Insulate from the ground, provide shelter and monitor vital signs carefully whilst awaiting rescue

You must not:

- Apply any form of cream, ointment or fat to the affected area
- Burst any blister that may form*
- Apply any form of adhesive dressing
- Remove anything that is stuck to the affected area

TREATMENT OF CHEMICAL BURNS

- Remove any chemicals from the skin by running the affected area under cool water for 20 minutes, or more. If the chemical involved is in powder form, such as lime, brush it off the skin before running the skin under water
- Remove any jewellery or clothing that may have been exposed to the chemical
- Apply a cool wet towel to help relieve pain or a large burns dressing if available to you
- Cover the burnt skin with a dry sterile dressing, or clean cloth
- If your casualty experiences an increased sensation of burning, rewash the skin for a further 10 minutes
- If the chemical burn is serious and impedes you evacuating to seek medical help, call the emergency services for assistance immediately

*See page 118 for the treatment of blisters

ELECTRICAL BURNS

Electrical burns can be caused by lightning or from a man-made source involving either, a high-voltage supply e.g. overhead power lines, or from a low-voltage supply as found in the home.

In all cases, an electrical injury can be life-threatening.

You may have multiple injuries to treat, including cessation of breathing, and a wound that enters the body as well as one that exits the body.

Your first priority is to ensure that it is safe to offer your casualty treatment.

In respect of a high-voltage injury, it is imperative that you and all bystanders stay well away from your casualty. Because the supply can 'arc', you must stay at least 18 metres away from the supply source.

You must call the emergency services immediately, detailing the extent of the incident.

In some cases of low-voltage injuries, the casualty may still have a contact with the supply, and therefore be 'live'. You must break the source of supply immediately before attempting any form of treatment. Switch the supply off from the main fuse-board. Failing that, remove the electrical device from the casualty. You can achieve this by standing on a dry insulating material and use a wooden or plastic object to drag away the source from the casualty ensuring that the area is safe for all.

As soon as you have deemed it safe to do so, you may start your treatment.

High-voltage injuries
- Keep everyone at least 18 metres away from the electrical source
- Call the emergency services
- Only when it is safe to do so, as directed by the emergency services, carry out your basic life support procedures

Low-voltage injuries
- Switch off from the MAINS supply if possible
- Break contact between the electricity and your casualty using an insulator, such as a piece of wood
- If you are unable to do this, you must insulate yourself before attempting to free your casualty from the supply

Once your casualty is free from the supply:
- Carry out your basic life support procedures
- Call the emergency services
- Be aware of any potential serious burns to deal with
- Insulate from the ground, provide shelter and monitor vital signs

Lightning strike

Only when it is safe to do so:
- Call the emergency services
- Carry out your basic life support procedures
- If they are not breathing normally, commence CPR
- Be aware of any potential serious burns to deal with
- Insulate from the ground, provide shelter and monitor vital signs
- Treat your casualty for shock
- If unresponsive but breathing normally, place them in the recovery position whilst awaiting rescue

BLISTERS

Blisters are small pockets of fluid that form on the skin in order to protect the underlying tissue from further damage. The friction motion causes the outer layer of skin to separate from the inner layers, leading to a sack of fluid building up in between to protect the area.

Blisters can develop anywhere on the body but the most common area in relation to outdoor first aid are the feet and hands, which occur due to the repetitive rubbing of the skin against the person's sock and footwear, or the friction from a rope against the palms of their hands.

Treatment

For a small blister, it is best practice to leave it alone and do not attempt to drain the fluid, as it should repair itself relatively quickly and will not impede on the activity.

For a medium-sized blister, you should apply a blister plaster which will offer protection to the area and provide a 'cushion' to reduce friction for when you continue with the outdoor activity.

For a large blister that is preventing you from continuing with the activity, apply a large gauze pad or general first aid dressing and tape in place. This will provide extra padding and support to either continue with the activity, or exit from the remote setting.

Draining a heel blister

If the blister is very large in size, you can drain the blister and then apply a blister plaster or dressing for protection. Although it is not recommended in workplace first aid, when you are in a remote setting it may be necessary so that you can evacuate your casualty without having to lift and carry them, or summon for professional medical assistance.

- Wear disposable gloves
- Clean the blistered area thoroughly using a sterile wipe
- Sterilise the needle by heating it with a naked flame until it is glowing red and then let it cool
- Insert the sterile needle into the outer edge of the blister
- Gently apply pressure on the blister using a sterile dressing or gauze pad to drain the fluid

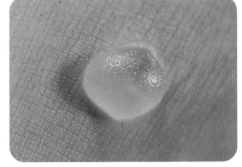

- Once the fluid has been drained, apply a sterile blister plaster or dressing to protect the area
- Leave the 'roof' of the blister intact which will act as an additional layer of protection for the affected area

Eye injuries have a number of different causes, such as a blow to the eye, foreign bodies, lacerations (cuts) and ultraviolet light. Eye injuries can also be caused by chemical exposures and burns as a result of liquid being splashed into the eyes.

A BLOW TO THE EYE

Serious and permanent eye damage can result from a blunt object, from a sports injury, a fall or being hit by a fist. Care should be taken when treating such an injury as the bone surrounding the eye could be fractured.

Signs and symptoms

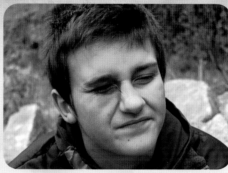

- Pain
- Swelling
- Bruising
- Possible bleeding
- Redness of the eye
- Blurred vision
- Headache

Treatment

- Gently apply an instant ice pack around the eye to sooth the pain and reduce swelling
- Offer your casualty a form of pain relief such as paracetamol or ibuprofen
- Treat your casualty for shock

Send your casualty to see their GP if:

- They have a change in vision
- The pain is persistent
- There is pus or warmth and redness, indicating infection
- They become forgetful or drowsy
- They have nausea, vomiting and/or dizziness
- The swelling does not subside after a few days

Go to your hospital accident and emergency department if:

- They have two black eyes (this could suggest a skull fracture)
- They have double vision
- They cannot move the eye
- They think something has pierced the eye
- There is a cut to the eye or blood inside the eye
- Fluid is leaking from the eye or the eye looks deformed
- They are taking blood-thinning medication such as aspirin, or have a bleeding disorder such as haemophilia

FOREIGN BODIES IN THE EYE

A foreign body in the eye is something that enters the eye externally from the body. Foreign bodies in the eye can cause minor discomfort, but can also cause severe damage, including loss of sight.

There are many foreign bodies in the outdoor environment which can cause damage to the eyes including wood splinters, soot from a burning fire, dust, dirt, debris, metal particles, bugs, insects and even a single eyelash can enter and damage the eye.

Signs and symptoms

- Sensation that something is in the eye
- Increase in tears produced by the eye
- Pain
- Blurred or double vision
- Sensitivity to light
- A visible foreign body on the cornea
- A rust ring or stain on the cornea if the foreign body is metal

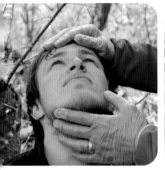 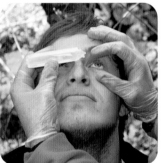 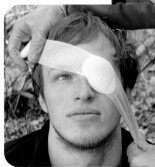

Treatment

- Wear disposable gloves
- Sit the casualty down, and stand behind them
- Lean their head back and very gently separate their eyelid with your finger and thumb and inspect the eye
- If you can see the foreign object, then try flushing it out with a sterile eye wash solution, or clean bottled water. Place a towel on the shoulder on the side of the injured eye. Lean the head back and inclined towards the injured side. Gently pour the eye wash into the eye to flush it out
- If this doesn't work, then you must seek medical advice

If there is something embedded, then you must leave it in place. Cover the eye with a sterile dressing, being extremely careful not to make any contact with the foreign body that is embedded. Transport them to hospital immediately, or summon for the emergency services for assistance.

LACERATIONS

Eye lacerations can be caused by making contact with sharp objects such as small tree branches, sharp plants such as gorse, flying objects such as grit, debris and shards of metal or glass.

Signs and symptoms

- Eye pain and sensitivity to light
- Increase in tears produced by the eye
- Blurred or distorted vision
- Squinting caused by spasm of the muscle surrounding the eye
- Feeling that something is in the eye and it cannot be removed

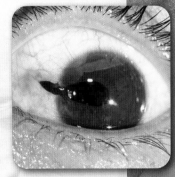

Treatment

- Wear disposable gloves
- Lie your casualty down and support their head in order to rest them. Try to keep both their eyes still
- Cover their injured eye with a sterile eye dressing, or ask them to hold a sterile dressing in place
- Insulate from the ground and provide shelter
- Take them to the hospital if you are able to evacuate the area and transport them. Failing that, call the emergency services for assistance

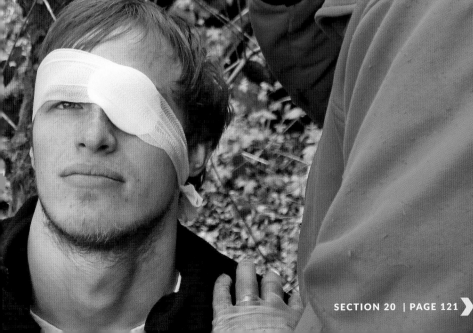

ULTRAVIOLET LIGHT

Ultraviolet (UV) light can lead to an eye injury called corneal flash burn.

Exposure to the sun can cause radiation damage to the eye, leading to flash burn. Damage is most likely to occur if you are in an arctic environment where the sun glares off snow and ice, or when you are at high altitudes.

Signs and symptoms

- Pain
- Redness and watering
- A gritty feeling
- Sensitive to light

Treatment

- Wear disposable gloves
- Cover the eye with a sterile eye dressing
- Take them to the hospital if you are able to evacuate the area and transport them. Failing that, call the emergency services for assistance

CHEMICAL BURNS TO THE EYES

The surface of the eye can be severely damaged with any type of chemical burn. It can lead to the loss of sight if it is not treated quickly.

Chemicals can be transferred to the eye by splashing, spraying or simply from your own finger should it be contaminated.

Substances such as insect repellent, fertilisers, pesticides, fuels and natural chemicals from plants can burn and damage our eyes.

Signs and symptoms

- Watering of the eye
- Pain
- Swelling
- Redness
- Evidence of the chemical

Treatment

- You must wear gloves to prevent yourself being contaminated by the chemical
- Irrigate the eye for 20 minutes under running cool water, or by flushing the eye with clean bottled water or saline solution
- Ensure that the irrigation does not flow into the other eye
- Try to identify the chemical so that the emergency services know what chemical they are treating
- Cover the injured eye with a sterile eye dressing
- Take them to the hospital if you are able to evacuate the area and transport them. Failing that, call the emergency services for assistance

POISONING

WHAT IS POISON?

Poisoning happens when you take into your body, a substance that damages your cells and organs, and injures your health.

Poisons are usually swallowed, but they can also be inhaled, splashed onto the skin or eyes, injected or received through a bite (as with snake bites).

Many substances are only poisonous if an abnormally large amount is taken. For example, paracetamol is harmless if you take one or two tablets for a headache, but is poisonous if you take an overdose.

A poison can enter the body in a number of ways:

- Swallowed; Food, alcohol, drugs etc.
- Absorbed; Chemicals, vapours etc. through the skin
- Injected; Drugs, medicine, stings etc.
- Inhaled; Gases, fumes etc.
- Splashed; into the eyes. Chemicals, etc.

General treatment for poisons

- **Call the emergency services immediately**
- **Place in the recovery position in order to maintain an open airway, and to allow vomit to drain from the mouth**
- **Keep any evidence of the poison to hand over to the emergency services**
- **Insulate from the ground and provide shelter**
- **Monitor vital signs and be prepared to resuscitate them**

DRUG POISONING

Recognition

Aspirin

- Upper abdominal pain
- Nausea and vomiting
- Ringing in the ears
- Confusion and delirium
- 'Sighing' when breathing
- Dizziness

Paracetamol

- Developing abdominal pains
- Nausea and vomiting

Tranquillisers (anti-depressants)

- Lethargy, sleepiness leading to unresponsiveness
- Shallow breathing
- Weak, irregular pulse

Narcotics

- Small pupils
- Sluggishness and confusion, possibly leading to unresponsiveness
- Slow, shallow breathing which may stop
- Needle marks which may be infected

Solvents

- Nausea and vomiting
- Headaches
- Hallucinations
- Unresponsiveness – possibly

Stimulants

- Excitable, hyperactive behaviour, wildness and frenzy
- Sweating
- Tremors
- Hallucinations

Treatment

- Protect yourself
- If responsive, place them in a comfortable position and try to establish the drug that has been taken
- Call the emergency services immediately
- Monitor vital signs
- Keep samples of vomited material and try to find evidence of the drug that was taken
- Be prepared to resuscitate them

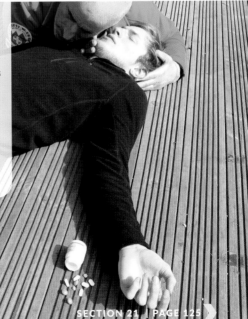

PLANT POISONING

Most plants that grow in the UK are harmless and, if eaten, may only cause a mild stomach upset.

If a potentially poisonous plant has been eaten, try to identify it so you can inform the emergency services, or take a sample with you to the hospital so that it can be identified.

The plants to look out for include, Wild Arum, Foxglove, Laburnum, Death Cap mushrooms, Ivy and Mistletoe - to name a few.

Recognition

- Nausea and vomiting
- Diarrhoea
- Impaired responsiveness
- Abdominal pains
- Seizures

Treatment

The same treatment can be applied as you would for drug poisoning (see page 125).

FOOD POISONING

This is usually caused by consuming contaminated food or drink. Some food poisoning is caused by foods that already have the bacteria in it, particularly from the E.coli or salmonella group of bacteria.

This particular poison could take hours or days before it takes effect.

The other main group are poisons produced by staphylococcus. The symptoms of poisoning develop far more rapidly, normally within 2-6 hours.

Recognition

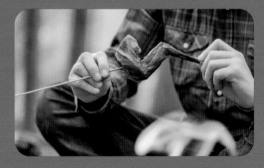

- Nausea and vomiting
- Abdominal pains
- Diarrhoea
- Fever
- Headache
- Impaired responsiveness

Treatment

- Encourage the casualty to rest
- Offer them plenty of bland fluids to drink
- Try to establish the source of the poisoning in case medical assistance is required
- Call the emergency services if their condition deteriorates

ALCOHOL POISONING

Alcohol poisoning results from drinking a toxic amount of alcohol, usually over a short period of time, which is known as binge drinking.

The intake of alcohol depresses the activity of the central nervous system, particularly the brain. Prolonged or excessive intake can severely impair all physical and mental functions and the casualty may become unresponsive.

Recognition

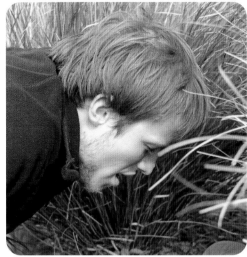

- Smell of alcohol
- Evidence of empty containers
- Impaired consciousness, leading to unresponsiveness
- Flushed appearance
- Deep, noisy breathing
- Nausea

In the later stages of unresponsiveness:

- Dry, bloated appearance to the face
- Shallow breathing
- Weak and rapid pulse
- Dilated pupils

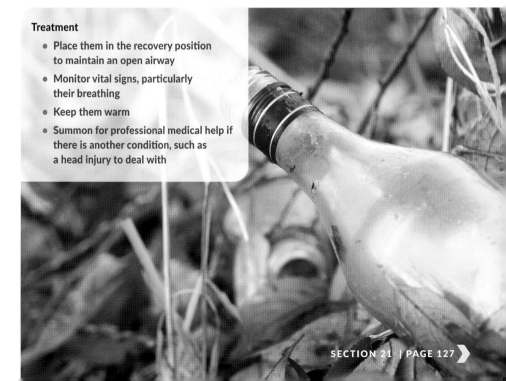

Treatment

- Place them in the recovery position to maintain an open airway
- Monitor vital signs, particularly their breathing
- Keep them warm
- Summon for professional medical help if there is another condition, such as a head injury to deal with

ANIMAL AND HUMAN BITES

Animal and human bites are a relatively common type of injury. In most cases, the wound that results from an animal bite is minor and can be treated with simple first aid techniques.

Dog bites

Dog bites typically cause a puncture wound in the skin. They can also cause a laceration and an abrasion. This is because dogs use their front teeth to "pin" their victim, and their other teeth to bite and pull at the surrounding skin.

Human bites

Most human bites are the result of a closed-fist injury, where one person punches another person in the teeth and cuts their hand. Typical symptoms include small cuts to the hand, and red, swollen and painful skin.

Treatment

The damaged body tissue following a human or animal bite is at risk of infection, especially in the outdoor environment, so you will need to treat your casualty immediately to reduce this risk.

Infections such as rabies and tetanus can occur following a bite, so your casualty will need to go to hospital for further examination and treatment to prevent these types of infection occurring.

- Make the area safe
- Reduce the risk of infection by wearing disposable gloves
- Inspect the wound for embedded objects such as teeth, and control the bleeding
- Thoroughly clean the wound and cover with a sterile dressing
- Treat for shock
- Evacuate to hospital if it is serious and the bleeding cannot be controlled

Symptoms of infection

- Redness and swelling around the wound
- The wound becomes more painful
- Discharge from the wound
- Swollen lymph glands (nodes)
- High temperature
- Shivers

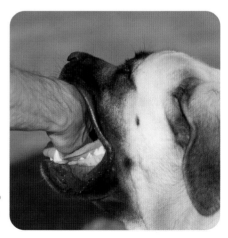

In cases of serious bites, where a body part such as a finger or ear has been bitten off, you should wash the body part with water and place it in a plastic bag or a sealed container. Put the sealed bag or container into another bag with instant ice packs surrounding the body part to keep it cool so that is can be transported to hospital - It may be possible to re-attach the body part using reconstructive surgery.

Do not freeze the body part or allow it to make direct contact with the instant ice packs.

SNAKE BITES

Snakes sometimes bite in self-defence if they are disturbed or provoked. Adders, or vipers, are the only wild venomous snakes in the UK.

Adders sometimes bite without injecting venom (toxins produced by the snake). This is called a 'dry' bite and may cause:

- **Mild pain caused by the adder's teeth puncturing the skin, and anxiety.**

If an adder injects venom when it bites it can cause more serious symptoms including:

- **Severe pain**
- **Breathing difficulties**
- **Swelling and redness in the area of the bite**
- **Nausea**
- **Vomiting**
- **Faintness**

Immediate action

If a snake bites you, or someone else, you should follow the advice listed below.

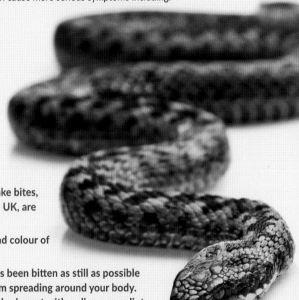

- **Remain calm and do not panic. Snake bites, particularly those that occur in the UK, are rarely serious and very rarely fatal**
- **Try to remember the shape, size and colour of the snake**
- **Keep the part of your body that has been bitten as still as possible because this will prevent the venom spreading around your body. You may want to secure the bitten body part with a sling or a splint. However, do not make the sling or splint so tight that it restricts blood flow**
- **Remove any jewellery and watches from the bitten limb because they could cut into the skin if the limb swells. However, do not attempt to remove any clothing, such as trousers**
- **Evacuate your casualty to hospital**
- **If your casualty's condition continues to deteriorate after treatment, call the emergency services for assistance**
- **If they become unresponsive, place them in the recovery position**
- **Insulate from the ground, provide shelter and monitor vital signs**

You should never:

- **Suck the venom out of the bite**
- **Cut the venom out of the bite wound with a knife or other instrument**
- **Rub anything into the wound**
- **Apply any tight bandage around the bitten limb to stop the spread of venom, such as a tourniquet or ligature**

INSECT BITES AND STINGS

Insect bites

Insect bites are a common occurrence in the outdoors, especially in the British summer months where we have a warm, wet and humid climate. Whilst most insect bites are more of a nuisance than harmful, some can produce painful side effects and the insect itself can carry infection.

After an insect bite, it is common to see a small red lump appear on the skin and the affected area may be painful and itchy.

Common insects found in the UK that bite include:

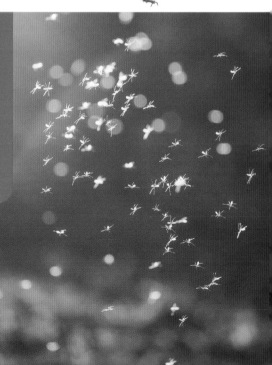

- Ticks
- Horseflies
- Midges
- Mosquitoes
- Fleas
- Mites

Insect stings

Many insects sting as a defence mechanism by injecting venom into the skin. In the UK, stinging insects include:

- **Bees** (honeybees and bumblebees)
- **Wasps**
- **Hornets**

If you are stung by an insect, such as a wasp, the area around the sting will become inflamed (swollen), go red and a raised mark (weal) will form. The affected area will often be quite painful and itchy. This will usually last for a few days.

People who have an allergic reaction to an insect sting will experience more symptoms. An allergic reaction occurs when the venom from the sting triggers the release of chemicals in the body, such as histamine.

Seek emergency medical treatment if, immediately after being stung, you experience any of the following:

- **Swelling or itching anywhere else on your body**
- **A skin reaction anywhere else, particularly pale or flushed** (red or blotchy) **skin**
- **Wheezing, hoarseness or any difficulty breathing**
- **A headache**
- **Nausea, vomiting or diarrhoea**
- **A fast heart rate**
- **Dizziness or feeling faint**
- **Difficulty swallowing** (dysphagia)
- **A swollen face or mouth**
- **Confusion, anxiety or agitation**

Treatment

Bee stings have a venomous sac attached. After you have been stung, the sting and the venomous sac will remain behind and the bee will die.

Wasps and hornets do not usually leave the sting behind and therefore could continue to sting you. If you have been stung and the wasp or hornet remains in the area, walk away calmly to avoid getting stung again.

Remove the sting immediately

As soon as you have been stung by an insect, you should remove the sting and the venomous sac. Do this by scraping it out with a hard edge, such as a plastic card or the blunt edge of a knife.

When removing the sting, be careful not to spread the venom further under your skin and that you do not puncture the venomous sac. Do not attempt to pinch the sting out with your fingers or a pair of tweezers, as you may spread the venom.

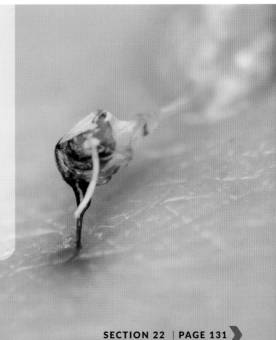

Basic treatment to treat bites and stings:

- **If possible, wash the affected area with clean water**
- **Put a cold flannel or a cold compress on the area to relieve pain**
- **Raise the part of the body that has been stung to prevent swelling**
- **Avoid scratching the area because it may become infected**
- **Monitor carefully for signs of an allergic reaction**
- **Visit your GP if the redness and itching gets worse or does not clear up after a few days**

TICK BITES

Ticks are tiny, eight-legged creatures that survive by feeding on the blood of animals and humans. Technically speaking, ticks are not insects, they fall into the same category as spiders - Arachnida.

Ticks can be found in areas with good vegetation, woodland and moorland areas across the UK and because of their tiny size, they can easily go unnoticed, even after they have bitten you.

Ticks are capable of transmitting infections such as Lyme disease, which, if left untreated, can cause severe, long term health problems.

Ticks can attach themselves anywhere on the human body, but mainly warm, moist areas such as the armpit or groin are targeted. Once a tick has found its way onto the body, it will bite into the skin and begin to feed. If the tick is not removed properly, the head and mouth parts can remain embedded and become infected.

If you have been bitten

REMOVE THE TICK AS SOON AS POSSIBLE!

- Wear disposable gloves
- Gently grip the tick using fine-tipped tweezers or a tick removal tool, getting as close to the skin as possible

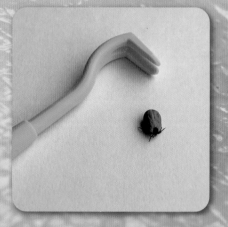
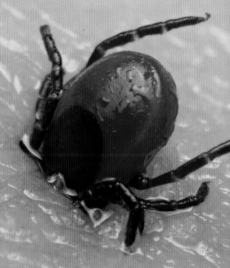

- Pull upwards very slowly and carefully without crushing the tick. If the head and mouth parts remain, the body will be susceptible to infection
- Once you have successfully removed the tick, wash your skin with clean water
- Apply an antiseptic cream to the skin around the bite
- Keep an eye on the bitten area for several weeks afterwards and if you begin to feel unwell, visit your GP

> DO NOT rotate or turn the tick using a tick removal tool, unless the manufacturer's instructions tell you to do so.